Asian
Aphrodisiacs

Other Books by the author

(Website:www.jerryhopkins.com
Email:jerry@jerryhopkins.com)

Bare Feet & Good Things to Eat (1965) with Gypsy Boots
You Were Born on a Rotten Day (1969) with Jim Critchfield
The Rock Story (1970)
Groupies & Other Girls (1970) with John Burks
Festival: An American Celebration (1970) with Jim Marshall &
    Baron Wolman (photographs)
Elvis: A Biography (1971)
The Last Sex Manual (1978) with Ron Pion, MD
No One Here Gets Out Alive (1980) with Danny Sugerman
The Hula (1981)
Elvis: The Final Years (1981)
Hit & Run: The Jimi Hendrix Story (1983)
Bowie (1985)
Fax to Da Max (1985)
Yoko Ono (1986)
The L.A. Book of Lists (1987)
Vinny, Part II, The Habilitat Story (1987) with Vincent Marino
Fax 2 Da Max (1988)
How to Make Your Own Hawaiian Musical Instruments (1988) with
    Martin Charlot (illustrations)
The Westin Maui (1989) with William Waterfall (photographs)
Kauai Lagoons (1990) with William Waterfall (photographs)
50 Simple Things You Can Do to Save Hawaii (1990) with Susan
    Manual
Frank DeLima's Joke Book (1991) with Frank DeLima
The Lizard King (1992)
The Jimi Hendrix Experience (1996)
Strange Foods (1999) with Michael Freeman (photographs)
Elvis in Hawaii (2002)
Extreme Cuisine (2004) with Michael Freeman (photographs)
In the Name of the Boss Upstairs: The Father Ray Brennan Story
    (2004)
Thailand Confidential (2005)
Bangkok Babylon (2005)
The Pacific Showman (2005) with Tom Moffatt
Asian Aphrodisiacs (2006)

Asian Aphrodisiacs

From Bangkok to Beijing–
The Search for the Ultimate Turn-On

Jerry Hopkins

PERIPLUS

Published by Periplus Editions (HK) Ltd, with editorial offices at
130 Joo Seng Road #06-01, Singapore 368357.

ISBN-13: 978-0-7946-0396-0
ISBN-10: 0-7946-0396-3

Printed in Singapore

Distributed by:

North America, Latin America & Europe
Tuttle Publishing
364 Innovation Drive
North Clarendon, VT 05759-9436
Tel: (802) 773 8930; Fax: (802) 773 6993
Email: info@tuttlepublishing.com
www.tuttlepublishing.com

Japan
Tuttle Publishing
Yaekari Building 3F
5-4-12 Osaki, Shinagawa-ku
Tokyo 141-0032
Tel: (03) 5437 0171; Fax: (03) 5437 0755
Email: tuttle-sales@gol.com

Asia Pacific
Berkeley Books Pte Ltd
130 Joo Seng Road #06-01/03, Singapore 368357
Tel: (65) 6280 1330; Fax: (65) 6280 6290
Email: inquiries@periplus.com.sg
www.periplus.com

09 08 07 06
 4   3   2   1

To my ever-patient wife, Lamyai

Contents

Chapter ten

Chapter eleven

Chapter twelve

Chapter thirteen

Chapter fourteen

Chapter fifteen

Chapter sixteen

Chapter seventeen

Chapter eighteen

Chapter nineteen

Chapter twenty

Introduction
Groucho & Me, On a Prowl

The *Lonely Planet* guide to Thailand calls Bangkok's weekend market at Chatuchak the "Disneyland of Thai markets," some eight thousand shops and stalls spread over thirty acres making its claim to be the world's largest open air bazaar a believable boast. It is a place where it's said you can buy anything—from hot meals, potted plants, kitchenware, arts and crafts, new and used clothing, to Buddha statues and magic amulets, furniture, fresh fruit and vegetables, and exotic pets, endangered ones if you ask discreetly and don't look like a cop.

So I was not surprised to find a man with a folding table selling aphrodisiacs. I picked up a bottle made from brown glass, about four inches high, approximately an inch in diameter. The label was in English as well as Thai and read: SKINK OIL WITH HERB INCEREASE PENIS SIZEL ADD HARD MAKES I GUARNTEE SALE FOR YOUR SPECIAL PURPOSE CERTAINLY 7 DAYS BY RMASSAGE. From which I gathered it was for external use rather than something to be consumed.

I was relieved to learn that because the word "skink" sounded familiar, but what, exactly, was a skink? I asked the vendor, a man about fifty wearing a baggy shirt and slacks, if I was correct.

"Same-same *jing jok*?" I said, using the Thai word for gecko. Was a skink a member of the lizard family?

His spoken English facility seemed even less equal to the challenge than the label on the bottle. Smiling, he said, "Four hundred fifty baht." A little more than $10.

I next looked at a jar no more than an inch high and an inch in diameter. Its label merely defined its purpose: GROW FOR HAIRY CREAM. Asians don't have much body hair and I guessed that along with a general wish to have lighter skin, there was a market composed of the non-hirsute.

"Two hundred baht," the salesman said.

That wasn't all. Along with the rows of small bottles and jars were flat boxes containing…I wasn't sure what. Picture a pale rubber band about the size of a coin with what looked like short stiff hairs about a quarter of an inch in length projecting outward from the perimeter.

I looked up at the vendor for guidance. "What's that for?" I asked, shrugging and turning my palms upward in what I hoped was the universal gesture for puzzlement. He smiled and mimed picking one up and fitting it over his penis. I bent forward and looked again.

Was it a cock ring? I guessed it was, but I'd never seen one that looked like that. Most were made from leather with a snap or Velcro to tighten it around the base of the cock. This looked like…suddenly I stood straight up. When I accepted the assignment to write this book, I sent an email plea to everyone I knew, asking for input and among the dozens of replies came one from a woman who told me about the dried eyelid ring of a sheep or goat (including the eyelashes). The dried ring was put in water to soften it, she said, then stretched open and placed on the penis just behind the head (not at the base) with the eye lashes upward. The idea being that the lashes tickled the lady's vagina as the man moved in and out.

I leaned forward and looked again. As far as I knew, there weren't that many sheep or goats in Thailand. And the eyelashes of a pig or water buffalo not only might be inappropriate, but also somewhat outsized, given the size of most local penises. (A subject I'll address soon.) I examined the product more closely, deciding that it, like so much for sale in Thailand, was counterfeit.

I returned my gaze to the "skink oil." I lifted the bottle and unscrewed the top, then raised it to my nose and sniffed. It smelled faintly reptilian—if something can smell slithery and somehow menacing—but who could tell for sure? As I screwed the top back onto the bottle, I asked myself: would I risk anointing my cock with this for seven days?

My reverie was interrupted as the vendor stated the price again, but this time it had come down a hundred baht. Recalling how many other things I'd done over the years with and to my genitals, I grinned and said, "Make it two hundred and fifty" and reached for my wallet.

Near the end of his fabled life, Groucho Marx was given an honorary doctorate at Harvard University and praised as a genius who contributed a new dimension to comedy, creating an original comic vocabulary and style. He acknowledged the critique with his trademark raised eyebrows and said every bit of the praise was well deserved and then he added that he would give it all back for "one more hard-on."

It was unfortunate that he didn't visit Asia, because when it comes to making it bigger, harder, longer-lasting and more fun, the men of the world's largest and most populous continent have been and continue to be more inventive and daring than their horny counterparts anywhere else.

And if Groucho had accompanied me on the journey I've taken around Asia, going where I've gone, swallowing the potions and pills that were guaranteed to make me "strong," doing what I've done to my genitals with lotions and mechanical devices and "toys"—his eyebrows would have gone up and down as never they had before.

He, like me, would have been amazed.

When my publisher suggested this assignment, he was too tactful to say so, but I knew he figured that I was suited for the quest. I was a skeptical Westerner who didn't believe in what I called "superstition." Tiger penis soup and rhino horn? Give me a break. Not only did men who consumed such things threaten the existence of two of the planet's magnificent creatures, the idea that they recharged one's sexual batteries seemed as ludicrous to me as it was environmentally incorrect.

Equally important was the fact that at age sixty-nine, like Hugh Hefner, who was a decade older, I was a fan of Viagra and other pharmaceutical wonders now part of what is called the "erectile dysfunction" (ED) marketplace.

Put simply, my cock no longer responded to my call as it once did and I found myself looking for help.

I'm also an old hippie who doesn't much care for chemicals, preferring (when I was a young hippie) peyote and hashish and marijuana to uppers and downers and LSD. And if I scoffed at much of the "alternative" medicine and therapies gaining a big following, I knew that numerous scientists in Europe and America were open to the notion that there might be real promise in the alternative health systems then making inroads in Western medicine than we doubters had surmised.

What's more, after researching and writing *Strange Foods* and *Extreme Cuisine*, two big books looking at what their titles implied, it was clear that I was willing to put just about anything into my mouth and swallow it. So when it came to exploring the world of aphrodisiacs, up close and personal, to my publisher it appeared that I had the balls for the job.

Finally, it further was my belief that life was for adventure…and that there was always time for one more. Thus researching and writing about Asian aphrodisiacs seemed a reasonable way to spend a year or two.

Call it a quest.

Call it a search for perfect sex.

Or, at least better than what I had last week.

And should there be any readers who think that I'm a male chauvinist pig, I plead guilty, but I also believe that if the preponderance of material on the subject of aphrodisiacs is male-focused, it may be because it's a phallocentric society we live in—and perhaps even more so in Asia than in the West—and it is he (not she) who has the bigger problem.

Say the word "aphrodisiac" and most people think you're talking about something to eat or drink. Some say it is something that has to "create desire, not improve performance and ability." That same source—*howstuffworks.com*—goes on to say some aphrodisiacs "create sexual desire by working on the mind, and there are those that create desire by affecting parts of the body. For example, something that increased blood flow in the sex organs might stimulate the feelings of sexual intercourse and have the effect of creating desire. Likewise, there are things that can make our bodies produce more of the chemicals associated with sexual desire. Something that lowers inhibitions in the mind, such as alcohol or marijuana, might also create (or allow) the desire to have sex. Sometimes, just thinking something is an aphrodisiac makes it appear to work as one."

Another authority, *Encyclopedia Britannica Online*, says an aphrodisiac is "any of various forms of stimulation thought to arouse sexual excitement" and divides them into two principal groups: "(1) psycho-physiological (visual, tactile, olfactory, aural) and (2) internal (stemming from food, alcoholic drinks, drugs, love potions, medical preparations)." This, too, remains somewhat vague, but it opens the door wide to interpretation.

In the chapters that follow, I meet the people, visit the places, and "road test" many of Asia's most popular aphrodisiacs. Following the *Britannica*'s lead, I include any substance, animal, vegetable, or mineral—and in the age of Viagra and its competitors, pharmaceutical—that is used to stimulate a man's or woman's libido, increase sexual energy, encourage and maintain the erection of the penis or increase feeling in the vagina and clitoris, intensify orgasm for all partners, and in any way possible enhance the enjoyment of sex. I further embrace belief systems such as Tantra and Tao; substances and mechanical devices for external and internal play (vibrators and cock rings and penis extenders and other toys, lotions, and aromatherapy); a variety of surgical procedures; music; and pornography that is used to win the same results.

This is not a book like any other about aphrodisiacs, and not just because I've gone with an expanded definition of what an aphrodisiac is. Go to *amazon.com* and you get hundreds of titles and from those I read, virtually all offer little but praise, most of them with a lot of strings attached. Quit smoking and alcohol and all recreational drugs, start an exercise program, change your diet (swear off fast food forever, etc.), and take these expensive pills two times a day for six months and, guess what, you'll feel healthier and probably sexier, too.

I don't see anything wrong with that. But it's not for me. Nor am I necessarily looking only for the quick fix. Let's face it, there's nothing growing on a vine or swimming in the sea or moving through the jungles that's going to produce the quick if temporary results of Viagra and a number of other chemical pick-me-ups that have been introduced in the past few years.

What this book is, then, is a look at the information that's come down through the ages about aphrodisiacs, with the focus on Asia, the region that has what I think is the most interesting history and greatest variety. Most of it is crapola, but some of it, after all this time, seems promising.

A Note about Geography

When embarking on this survey, I planned to include the Middle along with the Far East, as well as all the "stans" (Afghanistan, Kazakhstan, Turkistan, et cetera) and eastern Russia. But the outside world's notion of what is and isn't the Orient has changed. Where once Istanbul was regarded as the gateway to the East, now Turkey is knocking on the European Union's door. Including that vast part of the world also threatened to make this book overlong and unwieldy. So I decided to limit my study to what is more widely considered Asia today, stretching from the South (India, Sri Lanka, Bangladesh, Nepal, and Bhutan), across Southeast Asia (Burma, Thailand, Laos, Cambodia, Vietnam, Malaysia, Singapore, the Philippines, Indonesia, and Brunei), and northward to include China, Taiwan, the two Koreas, and Japan.

Chapter one
Rhymes with Niagara, Means the Opposite

Back in the 1980s, researchers at Pfizer & Company, an American pharmaceutical conglomerate that today is known for such popular over-the-counter remedies as Benadryl, Listerine, Neosporin, Rolaids, Sudafed, and Visine, as well as for numerous prescription drugs and animal health products, started looking for a class of chemicals with the potential for treating cardiovascular disease. The company began its research by examining hypertension, and that soon led them to angina, the chest and arm pain caused by poor blood flow to the heart. In the discovery process, Pfizer's chemists reportedly concocted about 1,500 chemical compounds, testing some for as long as four years.

In 1989, they found the chemical mix that we now know as Viagra and started clinical trials in the U.K. By 1992, results showed the medication to be not so wonderful as they'd hoped and the tests were stopped. That's when something unexpected happened. Men refused to return their test samples and some research subjects camped out on pharmacy doorsteps to see if they could get more of the stuff. It turned out that, as a side effect, Viagra gave erections to men who had long been suffering from impotence.

Pfizer hadn't become one of the world's largest pharmaceutical companies by being stupid, thus its chemists went full speed ahead with testing Viagra as something to treat erectile dysfunction, or ED. To everyone's delight, it turned out to be medicine's newest magic bullet, and the bedroom's Holy Grail. Not since the birth control pill was introduced in the 1960s had a medical discovery so completely changed the way many of the planet's inhabitants started relating to each other, as millions of flagging penises rose up like daffodils in the spring.

What Pfizer discovered was that their failed cholesterol drug suppressed the action of an enzyme that was responsible for breaking down nitric oxide. Nitric oxide (NO) had the effect of relaxing the walls of the capillaries, thereby allowing blood to flow freely into the penile shaft, engorge the tissues, and cause erection. As men get older, they produce less and less NO. Viagra reversed that process and got the blood flowing freely again, becoming the first oral medicine (a pill you take by mouth) that was proven to improve erections in a majority of men with impotence.

In 1998, after gaining approval by the Food and Drug Administration (FDA) in the U.S. and the European Union's equivalent, the European Medicines Evaluation Agency (EMEA), Pfizer found itself riding a wave of a size and force rarely seen in pharmaceutical history. This diamond-shaped blue pill became a cultural phenomenon—it seemed every issue of the *New Yorker* and *Playboy* had at least one cartoon—spreading around the world until, by 2004, Viagra was available in 123 countries, where more than twenty-seven million men had been treated by 600,000 prescribing physicians. Pfizer claimed on its website that nine Viagra pills were dispensed every second, nearly three hundred million tablets per year. In another statistic provided by Pfizer—reminding me of the signs we all used to see beneath the Golden Arches, tallying the number of world-wide burger sales—in the first six years, there were 1,066,102,768 tablets sold.

A billion new hard-ons! Think of it.

Okay, now here's the humorous side of the story. Pfizer insisted that Viagra was not an aphrodisiac.

When I discovered that Amal Naj, a onetime reporter for the *Wall Street Journal*, was the honcho for Pfizer in Thailand, Vietnam, Laos, and Cambodia, and was a fellow member of the Foreign Correspondents Club of Thailand, I requested a meeting and asked several questions. He did what men in his position likely do everywhere: he referred me to a "spokesperson" at the company's headquarters, in Pfizer's case in New York. Daniel J. Watts, with whom I then began an email correspondence, toed the company line voiced in early advertising stating: "VIAGRA is not a hormone, an herbal supplement, or an aphrodisiac. VIAGRA is a pre-scription medication that can improve the erectile function of most men with erection problems. So with VIAGRA, a touch or a glance from your partner can once again lead to some-thing more."

That sure sounded like an aphrodisiac to me, although I understood why it couldn't be marketed as such—especially in the West, where prevailing puritanical attitudes insisted that sex should be procreative and otherwise repressed.

Viagra came to Asia fast and within a year or two of its introduction, people started thinking it could have an unintended beneficial side effect: reducing the lethal pressure on some of the world's most endangered species. Viagra wasn't designed to have an environmental impact, but there was hope that its power to correct impotence might also reduce demand for various animal parts and plants that were consumed in the region as aphrodisiacs.

"For years," wrote Susan McCarthy in *salon.com*, "I've been hearing that rhinos—horribly endangered—are being slaughtered because Asian medicine prescribes rhino horn as an aphrodisiac. I've heard that tigers are nearing extinction because tiger bone is used in Asia as an aphrodisiac. I've heard that abalone, seahorses and sea turtles are also threatened by the same enormous demand for aphrodisiacs.

"So the advent of Viagra, the famous new erection-granting drug, made me wonder whether this would be a case of technology to the rescue. There was such a frenzy over Viagra in the U.S.—if there were even a fraction of that going on in Asian countries, might not people around the globe stop putting guns to the very heads of tigers and rhinos, turning on their heels and rushing down to the pharmacy?"

Susan was not alone in expressing such optimism. Frank von Hippel, who taught conservation biology at the University of Alaska, and his brother William, a professor of social psychology at the University of New South Wales in Sydney and a frequent customer at Chinese herbal shops in Hong Kong, published a hypothesis in *Science* magazine in 1998 and following three years of study, published positive results in the journal *Environmental Conservation*. They said sales had fallen in the market for sex organs of Canadian seals and reindeer antler—virtually all of which usually had been exported to China, Hong Kong, Taiwan, South Korea, and other parts of Asia. While *Time* magazine shouted on its May 11, 1998 cover the message, "Forget the deer tail, powdered seahorse, oysters on the half shell and candlelight dinners. There is a cure for IMPOTENCY and it's a pill called Viagra."

(A reporter conveniently named Bruce Handy wrote the story. He did not admit to trying Viagra, or any of the other ingredients, himself.)

Alas, it didn't mean much, as John Roach reported in *National Geographic News* soon afterwards that "Despite Prediction, Viagra Hasn't Stemmed Trade in Threatened Wildlife."

I wasn't surprised. For several reasons.

One: Many of the animal and plant "cures" for impotence appearing in what is called Traditional Chinese Medicine (TCM), in India's Ayurvedic medicine, in the Himalayas and Indonesia and elsewhere in Asia, and in the ethno-botany and folklore of just about everywhere else, were believed to salve or solve not just sexual problems but a variety of other maladies. Bear gall bladder and bile, for example, was hailed as an aphrodisiac, but also was used in TCM to treat a variety of illnesses including fever, convulsions, diabetes, and liver and heart disease. Similarly, tiger bone was thought to stimulate the libido, but it was also used to cure rheumatism, muscle pain, and paralysis.

Two: Superstition and folk belief die harder (and far, far more slowly) than Viagra and other pharmaceutical concoctions make any penis firm. The U.S. FDA declared that there was no scientific proof that anything sold over-the-counter (without prescription)—or, presumably, hunted and gathered in the wild—worked to treat sexual dysfunction. Still, a lot of people—mainly in Asia and in Chinatowns around the world—weren't listening.

Why? Simple. FDA's blanket condemnation clashed with "tradition" based on anecdotal evidence and ritual that had been handed down from generation to generation for millennia—TCM and Ayurvedic medicine dating back at least two and a half thousand years. Such traditions were not given up easily, because to surrender them would require the believer to admit that he or she was "wrong" and to abandon any hope that might be attached to those beliefs. And to deny any real benefit from the "placebo effect," the demonstrated good that sometimes comes from taking something that has no provable value.

In addition, the rarity of any species of fauna for which demand was high, especially in Asia, led to costs so high, the price itself often was regarded as evidence that they were the best possible "cures" available. A bowl of tiger penis soup might go for $350 in the black market in Hong Kong, South Korea, and Taiwan. Some consumers also purchased food and drugs made from endangered species as a show of affluence and of macho braggadocio.

Besides, even if the true believers had any doubts, so long as they could afford it, didn't it make sense to continue to use the traditional remedies and take Viagra or one of the other chemical compounds as well? What the hell could it hurt, except the endangered animal?

Three: Viagra and other prescription drugs were too expensive for most Asians, while the cost of most herbal remedies remained affordable. In 2006 in the pharmacy in Bangkok where I did my shopping, a package of four 100 mg Viagra pills cost $45, and its leading prescription competition Cialis cost $50, extravagant sums in a country where the minimum wage is under $4 a day.

This brings us to the subject of counterfeits. In the 1980s, the Itewan district in Seoul was one of Asia's first magnets for foreign shoppers looking for cheap knock-off goods. By the turn of the century, there were markets throughout Asia where copies of anything you wanted were available for an affordable price. In my neighborhood in Bangkok, credible copies of Rolex watches, top-of-the-line perfumes, the newest CDs and videos (including European, American, local, and Japanese pornography), designer clothing, computer software—were sold right on the street, and Asian countries led the world in the production of fake goods, including pharmaceuticals.

Much of this counterfeit medicine came from what could be called the "patent-free zones" of China and India. One copy, made in Mumbai, India, was called Kamagra, its name surely designed to evoke the *Kama Sutra*; in 2005, it was priced at $10 for four 100 mg pills, less than a quarter of the cost of Viagra. Another from India, called Zeagra, that I purchased in Cambodia, cost only $3! So, too, several "clones" from China. And, speaking from experience, they worked.

It's not surprising that Pfizer and other big drug companies in the West were not thrilled about this. Because these were not, in the legal sense, generic drugs. A generic drug— quoting America's FDA again—was a copy that was the same as a brand name drug in dosage, safety, strength, how it was taken, quality, performance, and intended use. The only thing that distinguished a copy from the "real thing" was usually the cost, with generics priced up to seventy per cent less than the identical compounds that carried the recognized brand names.

Generic drugs were less expensive because generic manufacturers didn't have the investment costs that the developer of a new drug had. Thus, new drugs were marketed under patent protection—the patent designed to safeguard this investment (including research, development, marketing, and promotion) by giving the developing company the sole right to sell the drug while the patent was in effect, usually a period of twenty years. Only as patents neared expiration, could other manufacturers apply to sell generic versions. Currently, almost half of the world's prescriptions are filled with generic drugs. And Viagra and *sildenafil citrate*, the chemical compound that is Viagra's active ingredient, isn't yet one of them.

Four: Governments in Asia have done nothing to promote the use of alternatives to products made from endangered species. While it is understandable that governments don't wish to be put in a position of endorsing herbal treatments and the like that haven't been clinically tested, it should also be pointed out that these nations also have, for a variety of reasons, failed to enforce existing laws about the killing and trafficking of these animals.

Five: My final reason for believing Viagra and all the others won't save the tiger, the rhino, the bear, and other threatened species is something I learned after I ran into a friend at a party and asked him if he'd met any interesting aphrodisiacs lately. (A conversational icebreaker guaranteed to work every time among Bangkok's aging expatriate community.) He said he'd purchased a bottle of something in Shanghai called Xingshijiu, supposedly made entirely from herbal ingredients. It was, he said, better than Viagra.

I went to good old Google and typed in the word Xingshijiu and learned that the Taiwan Department of Health had had a number of imported Chinese medicines tested. Xingshijiu was one of seven that were found to contain *sildenafil citrate*, the patented ingredient that made

Viagra work but was not naturally found in any of the herbs listed as ingredients. Another story, from Singapore, reported Xingshijiu was among three "herbal remedies" found to contain the same Pfizer chemical, again appearing in the bottled drink anonymously.

The obvious lesson being that you don't want to fight the enemy; you embrace him, add him (and it) to your recipe. In this fashion, ironically, Viagra didn't cut into sales of herbal remedies, it actually augmented them by increasing their effectiveness.

Chapter two
The Anatomy of Excitement

The body of evidence is not overwhelming, but what exists is in agreement: the Asian penis is smaller than those of Western men and men from the Middle East and Africa.

Many serious students of sex—from Alfred Kinsey in the mid–1940s to Masters & Johnson in the 1960s to the Janus Report in the 1990s—didn't consider size that significant, so they didn't care so much about its measurements as they cared about what men did with it. That said, in the small sampling the researchers did do, Asians always placed last, nearly an inch (2.5 centimeters) shorter than the average worldwide. A Caucasian penis averaged 6.4 inches (16 cm) in length, erect, while black males closely followed with 6.2 inches (15.5 cm). Hispanic men averaged 6.0 inches (just under 15 cm). And Asian men brought up the rear with 5.6 inches (13.7 cm). Some Internet webpages put blacks ahead of whites, but like so much information available in cyber-space, no recognizable or verifiable sources at the sites I found were identified. For the record, the longest on record (erect) was reported to be about 12 inches (30 cm), the shortest under half an inch (1.3 cm), not counting cases where men are born without.

More evidence was anecdotal. When I lived in Hawaii, where at least half the population was of Asian heritage, two sizes of condoms were sold in the pharmacies, marked on the packages "Regular" and "Oriental." Guess which ones were smaller.

Another story was probably apocryphal. Sometime during World War Two, or maybe it was the Korean War, America's propaganda geniuses suggested that condoms eight inches long (20 cm) be distributed behind enemy lines marked "Made in the USA—Small." I have not been able to find anyone to confirm this story, yet it remains a tale that begs the question: why would anyone make it up?

The important question is, does it really make any difference?

Ask the man who has one.

I don't know when people started measuring penises. Nowadays, all men do it. Is there a man reading this book who doesn't know the length of his cock? (It's measured from where the top of the erect penis meets the body, while holding it straight out, perpendicular to the torso. Not from beneath, which can add an inch or so.) The Kinsey Institute may say that "size is no more a measure of manhood, sexual capacity, or the ability to please a partner than is the size of a man's feet," as it did in a report in 1990, but many men disagree. Most men believe that size counts, and the problem is for many that it doesn't count high, or long, enough.

Before getting into the myriad things that Asian men do to increase their size, firmness, stamina, and pleasure (for their partners as well as themselves), we should consider the anatomy of a hard-on. For that is, after all, what much of this book is all about and it should be understood. Once acquainted with the basic physiology of the erection, it may be easier to comprehend and evaluate what is being offered on both the open and underground markets to enhance its appearance and performance.

And please, ladies, be patient. There is much here for you, too. Kinsey may have gone on to say there was "*no scientific research* suggesting that women generally prefer large penises, but there is research showing that most women *do not care* about their sexual partners' penis size." (Italics the Institute's.) Still, knowing what normally happens to the penis, however large or small, when a sexually attractive human comes into the horny man's view and/or imagination should be of interest to both sexes. In a moment, too, we'll take a look at what gets a woman excited, a subject about which most men probably are as dumb as a brick.

Okay, here we go, with a very short lesson in male anatomy.

Think of the penis as three hot dogs, two fat and one thin, running parallel, wrapped in a strong, fibrous and expandable sheath resembling a sausage skin (called the *tunica albuginea*) and topped by a small, helmet-shaped onion with a hole in it. The two fatter wieners, called *corpora cavernosa*, are next to each other on top and the thinner one, called the *corpus spongiosum*, nestles between and beneath. It contains the *urethra*, the thin duct that carries urine from the bladder, sperm from the testicles, and other precious bodily fluids from the prostate, Cowper's, and urethral glands. All three dogs are made up of erectile tissue and are inflatable.

Now picture the hot dogs with much of the contents removed. That's what the penis looks like when flaccid, or unerect. There are small arteries from the body leading to these hot dogs that are now dilated, reducing inflow of blood. In addition, there are small muscles down there that tighten to keep the hot dogs limp, so men don't embarrass themselves on the beach or in the office.

Okay. Now take that three-in-one hot dog into a go-go bar in Angeles City in the Philippines or show it some *anime*, the animated comic book porn that makes up such a charming part of the video market in Japan, or place it in a sexy setting with its owner's partner or new best friend anywhere from Jakarta to Shanghai to Mumbai.

If all goes well, desire assumes control, fantasies take flight, and messages from the brain go zipping down the spinal cord to the genitals, where several chemicals are released that relax the muscles, allowing blood to flow freely as the libido demands, simultaneously inflating all three hot dogs and the onion to capacity.

This is when it gets exciting, when the hot dogs become noticeable as an elongated bulge through a man's jeans and he begins thinking with what's called the "wrong head," as jokers say, the blood exiting the one on top of his neck to fill the one below his belt, often leaving the topmost one incapable of making a responsible decision but with a sappy grin on its face.

Judgment is suspended as the hot dogs almost double in diameter and length, due to the increased blood flow. The veins feeding the *corpora cavernosa* and *corpus spongiosum* when pumped up then are squeezed almost completely shut by the pressure of the bloated erectile tissue. The small muscles tense like rubber bands. The gates are closed! The blood cannot escape!

But of course that's not so for everyone. Millions of men can't get it up or maybe it goes only halfway or once there it goes quickly to sleep again. There are many reasons why.

Psychological explanations top the list, fear of failure being the most common, and in the list of diseases affecting a man's ability to get an erection, diabetes is the most common. It's estimated that up to fifty to sixty per cent of diabetic men are thus affected, tens of millions of them worldwide. Obesity is another cause and where once this wasn't a big problem, nowadays it's a growing one. Multiple sclerosis, bladder dysfunction, Parkinson's disease, stroke, and chronic kidney insufficiency add more.

Smoking and alcohol make things worse. Studies indicate that even two cigarettes will markedly decrease the blood flow to the penis if smoked before sex—and men who smoke two packs a day deflate faster, because the arteries as a long-term result constrict and harden. Alcohol attacks on many fronts, causing nerve damage, shrunken testicles, brain failure, and a rise in the female hormone, estrogen. And let's not forget that bit of Shakespearean wisdom about booze increasing desire while simultaneously reducing the capacity to do anything about satisfying it. How many cigarette smokers and heavy boozers are there in Asia? They are numerous.

More culprits are prescription drugs, especially some of those used by men with prostate cancer, diuretics, beta blockers and other drugs prescribed for high blood pressure and cardio-vascular disease, tranquilizers, and decongestants. No one knows how many men these affect, either.

The number of older men affected by the Limp Willy Syndrome for reasons of age is another unfathomable mystery. But it's estimated that as many as fifty per cent over the age of fifty are affected to some degree.

For me it did not seem promising. I drank—only beer, but in quantity. In 2000, I had had open-heart surgery—a triple bypass—and I was on a full complement of drugs to reduce my blood pressure and cholesterol level. And I was, alas, of a certain age.

The Lucky Lady's Anatomy

The female anatomy and its "requirements" during sex are both simpler and more complex, and surely deserving of more than a sidebar to the male's. Yet, as stated, the question of being better in bed is substantially more a man's problem than a woman's, as most women will attest.

The vagina is a pink, tubular hallway about four inches (ten centimeters) long and about an inch (two and a half cm) wide that takes the visitor from the vulva and fleshy lips on the outside to the uterus on the inside. This is where much of the fun occurs. This also is the path for menstrual fluids leaving the body and the elastic channel through which a baby is born.

It is the elasticity that allows objects far larger than the relaxed dimensions here stated might indicate. Just as a man's little worm may, on excitement, become a fence post, the vagina may become a orifice into which the fence post comfortably fits. This is most easily accomplished when glands near the vaginal opening and the cervix release a woman's natural lubrication. More liquid may seep through the vaginal wall.

For some women this doesn't always happen so easily. Some men are so randy they may be turned on by a Victoria's Secret catalog (in my youth, it was Sears Roebuck), but for many women it often takes a greater effort or commitment from both sides of the bed. Still, for sexual intercourse to occur, the woman doesn't have to "get it up" and keep it there. In this way, sex may seem "easier" for the female than the male, although that's probably a male point of view.

What leads a woman to sexual pleasure, or orgasm? There are nerve endings close to the entrance of the vagina, not unlike the nerve endings in the man's penis. Equally important, at the opening of the vagina is the clitoris, a bump often compared to the penis because it becomes larger and more erect when the woman is sexually excited. Gentle friction here usually delivers pleasure, too.

Finally, about two inches (five cm) inside the vagina (for some but not all women) is the legendary "G-spot," which can produce intense orgasm if stimulated in a way that suits the individual.

Chapter three
Aphrodisiacs from 400 B.C.

India might not be as much fun today as it was back when the *Kama Sutra* was first compiled in Sanskrit from more than a dozen ancient texts, when in the fourth century AD, a Brahman scholar named Vatsyayana explored the connection between mystic experience and amorous Ecstasy. In the centuries that followed, his text was well received, and the numerous and imaginative positions of sex described in the book were artistically carved in stone and graphically displayed on Hindu temple walls over much of India.

In this fashion, what purportedly described the sexual mores of cultured Hindus became a sort of "chapbook," first for the population of the great subcontinent and later, in the twentieth century, when it became a sex manual for the Love Generation in the West. With the introduction of the birth control pill in the early 1960s and the "sexual liberation movement" that quickly followed, the pages devoted to "sexual congress" that read somewhat like a handbook for Chinese acrobats became the world's most widely known guide to the pleasures and techniques of sex.

Ironically, by that time in India, the sexual tide had reversed, thanks in large part to Victorian era Anglo-Saxon prejudice. Mahatma Gandhi, educated in England, is justly revered as the guru of modern India's spirit and spirituality, but what isn't generally remembered is that he dispatched his disciples in teams to smash erotic temple art. And as Alain Daniélou stated in the introduction to his translation of the *Kama Sutra* (published in 1994), Pandit Nehru, hailed as the true father of what we know as India today, "was irritated by my having photographed and published the photographs of sculptures showing homosexual relations, dating from the eleventh century, when he claimed that such vice in India was due to Western influence." It was Nehru, too, who pushed through laws forbidding anal and oral sex "with a man, woman or animal." Daniélou observed, "The country of the *Kama Sutra* had thus been relegated to the level of the most backward countries in the sphere of liberty."*

It was in the holy city on the Ganges called Benares (since renamed Varanasi) that Vatsyayana collected the ancient manuscripts from which he drew his inspiration and quoted numerous important passages. When I visited Varanasi more than 1,600 years after Vatsyayana, I stayed in a guesthouse overlooking the Ganges and the *ghats*, the wide riverside platforms with steps that led directly into the river. Varanasi had been continuously populated for three thousand years, making it a contemporary of Thebes and Babylon. This also was Shiva's sacred city and that made the waters especially powerful. Every Hindu at some time in his or her life, if possible, made a pilgrimage here, more than a million every

---

* The *Kama Sutra* will be quoted in several chapters, sometimes from other translations, and which version will not always be identified.

year, coming to purify themselves with a dip at dawn.

I had missed the early crowds when I walked the mile or two into the old city center my first morning in the ancient city, but still there were many dressed in loincloths or translucent white garments, submerging themselves and pouring the water over their heads, even drinking it, while praising and imploring the multitudinous Hindu gods. Here and there, too, were some of India's famed *sadhus*, the naked holy men who invented dreadlocks centuries before Bob Marley stopped combing his hair, their bodies painted in bold colors, carrying tridents and human skulls, and smoking *ganja*, another taste that long predated that of the Jamaican reggae king.

I passed a dozen men hosing away a thick accumulation of silt from the upper steps, deposited by seasonal flooding from the melting Himalayan snow hundreds of miles to the north. As the stone stairways returned to view, women moved in and draped them with saris and guesthouse laundry and bedding they had just washed in the river, to dry quickly in the scorching sun. Here, as well, wandering cows left their pungent deposits and more women formed the manure into large pancakes, to be used after drying as a fuel for cooking.

Today the Ganges is one of the most polluted rivers in Asia, but I was assured the crowds increased every year, as Varanasi was India's Jerusalem, the Moslem faith's Mecca. To die in Varanasi, was to achieve *moksha*, to escape the eternal wheel of reincarnation and be transported into Shiva's arms in heaven. This occurred at the "burning *ghats*," where open cremations were staged around the clock, the untouchable Doms, the lowest of India's castes, cutting and splitting an endless supply of wood and supervising the fiery passage to paradise. Flower petals and powdered sandalwood were sprinkled over the corpses and when the ashes cooled (up to three hours later), the remains were sprinkled on the holy river below. If the deceased couldn't afford the fees for this service, they were wrapped in cloth and merely set adrift. Infants and children were not cremated, either, as they were regarded as innocent; instead they were taken out in boats, their small bodies weighted with rocks, and sunk.

Anywhere else on the planet, riverfront real estate would long have been usurped by developers, but Varanasi seemed to be the exception to all such rules. Some of the low-rise buildings closest to the river were converted into guesthouses, like mine, and souvenir stalls nearby offered a variety of lurid postcards and cheaply produced replicas of the *yoni* and *lingam* statues seen in every Indian village square, guaranteed to produce giggles back in the U.S. or the U.K. But when I entered the old city, it was to disappear into a labyrinth of alleys too narrow for sunlight to reach the ground or two large holy cows to pass, a neighborhood that reeked of the past.

Merchants in tiny storefronts sold lacquerware and brass pots, lotus flowers and red tilak powder, saris in a hundred hues. Teashops with stained plaster walls and low stools and tables served *ganja* cookies and pastries adorned with silver foil. Bags of curry powder and medicinal herbs added their scents to those of burning incense, garbage, mildew, urine, and manure. There were motorbikes in the alleyways and small children wore tee shirts bearing the names of European rock and roll bands, but I felt as if I might encounter Vatsyayana at any turn.

For nearly an hour I wandered aimlessly—easy to do as there seemed to be no plan to this urban honeycomb—and after stopping for tea and cookies and outpacing the last of too many persistent "guides" and touts, for which India is infamous, I finally exited the maze and with considerable relief came upon a bookshop with a single clerk.

"Do you have any copies of the *Kama Sutra*?" I asked.

With a slight bow, he told me he did and asked if I'd heard of the *Ananga Ranga*? "It's another fine old text," he said, leading me to the rear of the shop. "We also have copies of *The Perfumed Garden*, from Arabia. You are a student of the sex?"

His English was schooled, almost scholarly, the words emerging in the charming Indian fashion that sounds a bit like water boiling.

We halted before some shelves that ran from the floor to the ceiling, from which he extracted a large book called *The Erotic Art of India*.

"You will enjoy this," he said, his eyebrows rising and falling twice, reminding me of my inspiration, Groucho Marx.

Half an hour later I left with four different editions of the *Kama Sutra* and several other volumes extolling in picture and prose the failure of Gandhi's goons in their effort to wipe out the country's erotic past, some of the photo books depicting the numerous erotic carvings and monuments that survived, the best display of them in a temple complex a two-hour plane flight away. I planned to go there on the weekend.

That night in my guesthouse, following a vegetarian supper, I turned the pages of some of the translations of the *Kama Sutra*, learning that there were three types of men according to their genital size: the rabbit type (small), the bull (medium), and the horse (large). Three different animals were used to type women, depending on the depth of their respective vulva: deer, cow, and (I'm sure it wasn't meant as an insult) elephant. Vatsyayana went on to say that there were three equal unions between persons of corresponding dimensions (rabbit/deer, bull/cow, and horse/elephant) and six unequal ones (rabbit/cow, rabbit/elephant, bull/deer, bull/elephant, horse/cow, and horse/deer).

"The woman places herself on all fours on the ground in the posture of the cow ready for the bull's assault. This is the position of The Cow," Vatsyayana advised. "In the same fashion, one can imitate other animals, mounting the woman like an ass, playing with her like a cat, attacking like a tiger, stamping like an elephant, pawing the ground like a pig, riding horse-fashion. Thus one learns a thousand ways to copulate."

I was told also to mimic the insect world. (Think about that the next time you watch the Discovery Channel.) There were four kinds of mild embrace and four more that were more vigorous, five kinds of kisses, eight kinds of oral intercourse, and nine ways of moving the *lingam* inside the *yoni*. Everything from sex with several women (called The Herd of Cows) to male and female homosexuality to bestiality to adultery to transvestism to violence was described and approved.

There were sections on "The Art of Scratching" and "Biting," not playfully, but seriously, drawing blood and leaving marks. "There are four ways of hitting," it was advised in the chapter called "Blows and Sighs," "—with the side of the hand, with the palm of the open hand, with the fist, with the ends of the fingers joined. The woman groans under the blows, because they hurt her." This chapter concluded with a warning: "One must in all cases know when to stop if there is a risk of mutilation or death."

For many readers today, such advice was as sexist as it may have been sexual. It's true that women were told how they could get money from men, but always they took a submissive role in doing so. "Vigor and audacity are manly qualities," Vatsyayana wrote. "Weakness, sensuality, and dependence are female characteristics."

The young men and women on the old hashish trail that led from Europe through Turkey and Afghanistan and to the beaches at Goa on India's west coast, then north through Benares to Kathmandu, with a visit to an ashram somewhere along the way to chill out, may have fancied themselves liberated, but the text many said they admired (and may never, in fact, have read) was not.

Yet, it suited the time of its compilation, when Hinduism, so class- and color-conscious, espoused behavior not only aimed at satisfying religious, social, and moral obligations, but also material comfort (*artha*) and sexual pleasure and love (*kama*). In Reay Tannahill's superb *Sex in History* (1992), the author called *artha* and *kama* "the sugar on the pill of sanctity. But they were sanctified just the same. Sex, for the Hindu Indian as for the Taoist Chinese, was a religious duty—not one that would put him straight into tune with the infinite, but certainly one of the least taxing and most pleasurable ways of improving the state of his *karma*."

My interest in the *Kama Sutra* was drawn to the text's final pages where there were sections dealing with "tonic medicines" and "ways of enlarging the *lingam*...miscellaneous experiments and recipes." A few were simple and sounded harmless, however dubious. For example: "Mix garlic root with white pepper and licorice. When drunk with sugared milk, it enhances virility." Another said a man "who wishes to copulate during a whole night, and whose desire, having come on suddenly...must get a great number of eggs, so that he may eat to excess, and fry them with fresh fat and butter; when done, he immerses them in honey, working the whole mass well together. He must then eat them as much as possible with a little bread, and he may be certain that for the whole night his member will not give him any rest."

It was advised that boiling a goat's testicles in sugared milk would accomplish the same thing. In another recipe, I was assured that "camel's milk mixed with honey and taken regularly develops a vigor for copulation which is unaccountable and causes the virile member to be on the alert night and day."

Was this really the way the Hindus lived fifteen hundred years ago? I took a plane to Khajuraho, a dusty village in the middle of nowhere that fortunately was served by the national airline in daily flights that went from Delhi to Agra (where the Taj Mahal is located) to Khajuraho to Varanasi, and back again. Khajuraho was on this esteemed route because twenty-four temples situated there of an original eighty-five were among the world's greatest temples of love, where handsome men and extraordinarily voluptuous women and more than a few strong animals brought the *Kama Sutra* to life, or at least to stone. Nowhere on earth, outside of a porn shop in San Francisco, had I witnessed sex depicted with such frankness and variety…and in India, unlike in California, sex had been rendered art.

Khajuraho—now a small town of about 7,000—was once the religious capital of the Chandela Rajputs, a Hindu dynasty that ruled this part of India from the tenth to the twelfth centuries. The temples, now listed as a UNESCO World Heritage Site, were built over a span of a hundred years, from 950 to 1050 AD. Then, like the larger Khmer temple complexes in Cambodia, they were abandoned to the engulfing jungle until rediscovered in 1838 by a young British engineer, T.S. Burt, who said in his report: "I found…seven Hindoo temples, most beautifully and exquisitely carved as to workmanship, but the sculptor had at times allowed his subject to grow a little warmer than there was an absolute necessity for his doing: indeed some of the sculptures here were extremely indecent and offensive, which I was at first much sur-prised to find in temples that are professed to be erected for good purposes, and on account of religion. But the religion of the ancient Hindoos can not have been very chaste, if it induced people under the cloak of religion, to design the most disgraceful representations to desecrate their ecclesi-astical erections." I will assume that last phrase was a slip of Mr. Burt's facile tongue.

Apparently, no one really knows why the carvings are so erotic. The Chandelas barely mentioned the temples in their literature. Some say the carvings were inspired by the *Kama Sutra*. Others linked them to Tantric cults that used sex as a part of their worship or to honor and appease the gods, so that the city would be spared from natural disaster. Another explanation came from the Indian scholar Shobita Punja, who wrote in her book, *Divine Ecstasy* (1992), that the sculp-tures represented the marriage of Shiva and Parvati and the subsequent orgy that may have matter-of-factly followed such heavenly events.

Mr. Burt was, of course, a man of his culture and time. When I arrived in Khajuraho a hundred and fifty years later, I confess that I found everything just as I wished it had been in my Protestant temples of worship in the U.S. when I was growing up but, alack and alas, was not.

Chapter four
Ayurvedic Medicine: Going to Bed with the Gods

Sex in India may not appear to be as much fun nowadays, or as bizarre as it was in the period leading up to the publication of the *Kama Sutra* and the construction of the erotic temples. Yet however conservative Hindu society has since become, it clearly remains in the lead in the prescription of herbal aphrodisiacs, going so far as to suggest that anyone having a sexual relationship should be taking aphrodisiacs on a regular basis, not only to make sex more satisfying but also to maintain the overall health of the body and prevent general health problems.

Such advice is a part of Ayurveda (pronounced ah-yer-vay-duh), the ancient system of medicine that encompasses a range of treatments including herbs, lifestyle and dietary modification, meditation, massage, yoga, breathing exercises, cleansing measures such as nasal douching and enemas, prayer, aromatics, and to a lesser degree astrology, gems, amulets, and color to maintain or restore health. As such, it obviously not only differed from western medicine—which until recent years treated disease rather than considered steps to prevent it—it also was based upon the need to maintain a balance between three varying types of bodily energy that controlled various physiological functions and reflected certain physical body types.

Like many "natural" or "traditional" medical systems, Ayurveda originated in myth. In this case, untold thousands of years ago, according to the sacred Hindu text *Ramayana*, a god named Lakshmana, brother of the all-powerful Rama, lay dying. His faithful deputy Hanuman, the monkey god, was dispatched to a holy peak in the Himalayas to harvest life-saving herbs, but uncertain which ones to bring back, he lifted the entire mountain and carried it to his master. On the way, numerous plants fell off, scattering across the land and taking root. In this fashion, Ayurdevic science was given to all of India, the thousands of consequent herbal remedies thus arriving as a gift from the gods.

Ayurveda is Sanskrit for what usually is translated to mean "science (or knowledge) of life," and it is defined by the belief that health results from harmony between mind, body, and spirit. (A not uncommon belief shared by a growing number in the developed world today.) The theory is that we are born with our energies, or *doshas*, in balance, and when that balance is upset, we need to do something about it.

There were, it was said, "qualities of nature" called *gunahs*, the opposites found in all nature and human activity: heavy vs. light, slow vs. quick, cold vs. hot, wet vs. dry, smooth vs. rough, solid vs. liquid, soft vs. hard, stable vs. mobile, subtle vs. gross, and non-slimy vs. slimy. In addition, there were five "great elements," called *punchamahabhuta*, that combined to form the material world: ether, air (or wind), fire, water, and earth. These, in turn, were reduced to three main "medical humors," or *doshas*: *Vata* (air), *Pitta*, (fire), and *Kapha* (water), each favoring particular body types and, thus, tending to dominate—*Vata* for those with lighter frames, either short or tall and thin, individuals with dark hair and eyes, creative and imaginative souls with fears, anxieties, and insecurities; *Pitta* fitting the generally average physique, accompanied by lighter hair and eyes, more intellect and anger; *Kapha* being sturdier and thicker, slower but steadier and calmer, yet greedy and possessive. The three *doshas* were also connected to different bodily functions—*Vata* controlling blood flow, waste elimination, hearing and speech; *Pitta* heat, metabolism, digestion, sensory perceptions, and discrimination between right and wrong; *Kapha* lubricating the joints, healing wounds, giving biological strength, supporting memory retention, maintaining immunity.

There's more, but you can see why many in the West threw up their hands. That said, it should also be pointed out that before the nineteenth century and the discovery of bacteria and viruses along with a greater understanding of cellular structures and organic chemistry, the West was pretty clueless, too. Not so long ago in the developed world, superstition and trial and error characterized most medical treatment everywhere.

Thus, when the British began to establish western styled hospitals and introduced the start of a national health service, Ayurveda was not included. The principles of Ayurvedic medicine may have been around for millennia longer than those developed from the time of Hippocrates, and its practitioners correctly claimed it was one of the oldest systems in the world—dating back 2,500 to 5,000 years; scholars differ— but Western medicine consistently pointed to the fact that few of its potions and principles had been tested and proven to have any genuine effect.

As noted, many of the herbal remedies prescribed were aphrodisiacs, called *Vajikarana*, a *vaji* being a horse. These were the substances that gave the power or vitality of a horse, particularly the animal's great capacity for sexual activity. It should be noted by my female readers, that in the equestrian world there are mares as well as stallions.

Carroll Dunham is an American expatriate who operates a company called Wild Earth in Nepal that produces herbal products for export (her clients include the international chain of Body Shops), a woman often called by her friends the "Ruth Westheimer of the Himalayas," a reference to the peppery, media-wise American sexologist known as Dr. Ruth. Carroll wants it made clear that Ayurvedic "cures" are not in competition with Western ones.

"The herbal argument always is that it works more slowly for chronic conditions, but for longer lasting results," she told me. "In other words, if you take *ashwagandha* mixed with some twenty other herbs over a six-month period, rather than take Viagra, it will take longer before you see results but the results will last longer and you will have far fewer side effects. Most people," she said, "don't have the patience."

Carroll, who also organizes women's groups in Nepal to harvest and export the herbs, further distanced herself from the West when she said, "Many of the physical substances you will find in aphrodisiac texts are related to states of mind and shifting consciousness, not just creating hard-ons. The point is union and when energies properly flow, pleasure melts internal places, and new places open for surrender and energies build and mount, intensity rises and flows in a deeper way than the mechanical following of some sex manual."

The European Institute of Vedic Studies in Sauve, France, took a somewhat less ecstatic view, but adhered to the holistic dictum that while in the West "aphrodisiac" often meant "to arouse the sexual organs," in Ayurveda the same word meant "that which strengthens the body by reinvigorating the sexual organs." A strong *shukra*—the sperm of the man and the ovum of the woman or their potential to create life—will help protect both sexes from diseases of the genitals, the Institute said in an article called "The Ayurvedic Understanding of Aphrodisiacs" (2004), and "the daily use of aphrodisiac herbs over a period of a month or several months will increase the capacity for a couple to enjoy love-making for longer periods of time."

Further support of Ayurvedic herbs is in the prevalence of plant use in medicine worldwide. An estimated eighty-five per cent of the world's population goes to herbalists of one type or another for their primary healthcare. Some may argue that that's because their choices are skewed economically or culturally in that direction, but it should also be noted that as many as forty per cent of the pharmaceuticals in use in the West currently contain plant-derived materials or synthesized ingredients from agents originally taken from plants—including, for example, mint (a natural source of menthol), opium and coca (for morphine and other painkillers), cinchona (quinine), et cetera.

The following plants are not well known in the West as aphrodisiacs, but perhaps some day they will:

Ashwagandha (*Withania somnifera*) has been popularized as India's most potent "hot plant" and sometimes has been called "India's ginseng," a reference to the plant that wins highest praise for its sex-enhancing powers in Traditional Chinese Medicine. Some translate its Sanskrit name as "he who is as virile as a horse," still another reference to an animal that conveys a clear image of strength yet plays a small role otherwise in India's modern society.

It is used in a number of forms (powdered, in an oil or

poultice, et cetera), as nerve tonic, rejuvenator, and calmative, as well as to treat an endless list of ailments, ranging from sexually transmitted diseases to the common cold to leprosy, but it is best known as a stamina-enhancing herb and as a powerful aphrodisiac.

It's a tough little plant, a small woody shrub that requires little care or irrigation, even in the dry parts of southern India. Its long taproot and mass of smaller roots, when dried, yield about seventy kilograms (one hundred and fifty pounds) per acre once a year, and because of its popularity, vast fields are dedicated to its cultivation. Some sources say it's mainly for men, others say it serves both sexes.

Lakshmana (*Convolvulaceae*) is named for the Hindu god credited with spreading Ayurvedic science across India. This is a vine with heart-shaped leaves and a blossom called the Shiva tendril. Christian Räatsch wrote in *Plants of Love: The History of Aphrodisiacs and a Guide to Their Identification and Use* (1997), that *lakshmana* is considered "a yoga plant and symbolized the *kundalini* serpent, that active female energy that links humans with the divine. According to yogic philosophy, every person carries such a serpent in his or lower abdomen. When it is fed, it awakens the sexual powers."

Datura (that's the Latin name), which translates as "divine inebriation," is generally known as the thorn apple; four of its ten species are indigenous to South Asia. All play a role not only in traditional medicine but in psychotropic drug use, the latter effect so pronounced that Richard Schultes (modern history's most famous botanist in the field, famed for his work in the Amazon and Mexico) and Albert Hofmann (inventor of LSD) together said there was no need to ask why primitive peoples considered them "plants of the gods."

Its alkaloid-rich seeds and leaves frequently were combined with hemp, opium, small pieces of betel and spices. It then was smoked, eaten, drunk, or taken as an enema. Carroll Dunham said it was "blown up the anus of a couple in sexual embrace to help enhance states of deeper awareness. Think," she wondered, "who has that job!" Most commonly, she added, its leaves were steeped as a tea or its seeds soaked in alcohol and its use was "really all about transforming perception rather than enhancing the sexual act."

Asafetida (*Ferula asafoetida*) is a type of fennel that grows to sometimes twelve feet (four meters) in height and is called "Devil's Dirt (or Dung)," a reference to its sulphurous smell and garlic-and-onion taste. It is regarded as one of the stronger Ayurvedic herbs, consumed to aid digestion, as an antispasmodic and expectorant, and to calm nervousness.

The active ingredient when taken as an aphrodisiac is found in the milky sap within the turnip-like root, fibrous stalk, and leaves. This hardens into granules upon contact with the air and may also be used as a spice when cooking. Usually it is stir-fried to remove a natural irritant or dried and taken in capsule form, alone or mixed with equal parts of ginger, black pepper, long pepper, ajowan, cumin, black cumin, and rock salt.

In Tibetan medicine, which shares many of the same herbs with Ayurveda, it is often referred to as the No. 1 aphrodisiac.

Bala (*Sida cordifolia*) literally means "strength," the presence of a number of active alkaloids (including ephedrine) believed to rejuvenate and strengthen the body. The leaves are used as an infusion in treating fevers and in delirium, the root is used.

Shatavari (*Asparagus racemosus*) reverses the harem concept of ancient India and translates as "she who has one hundred husbands" and I suppose it should be assumed, therefore, that she who consumes it has the capacity to make love almost endlessly, although substantiating reports are lacking.

More realistically, it is one of the best-known rejuvenating tonics for women, with similar effects to *ashwagandha's* action on men, though both are active for each sex. It is a rich source of Vitamin A, hence it has been used to treat eye disease. It is traditionally grown in terracotta pots and used as a salad vegetable and in candied sweets.

Kumari (*Aloe vera*) is one of the best known and most widely accepted medicinal plants in the world, a spiky succulent that is so effective in treating burns and other minor skin injury that it appears not only in various forms in hospitals and doctors' offices worldwide, but also in many commercial sunscreen products, as well as in shampoos and beauty creams.

There are many advocates who make it sound as if it were India's answer to whatever it is that Madonna puts in her morning cup of tea, its meaning translated as "like a young girl or virgin," bringing the energy and stamina of youth to the female reproductive system. While it is true that the plant contains more than seventy-five nutrients and twenty minerals, nineteen amino acids, and twelve vitamins, such claims are, so far, unproved.

Cotton (*Gossypium herbaceum*) is one of the most widely used plants in the production of textiles and is grown in many parts of the world. Not so widely recognized are the essential oils obtained from the seeds and the resins and tannins extracted from the root. It is the latter that find a use in Ayurvedic medicine in a rejuvenating drink believed to have aphrodisiacal qualities.

It's not clear whether or not these plants will make their way onto western drug store shelves and those that do, likely will be synthesized because the replacement of herbs with synthetic drugs—a relatively new phenomenon, less than a century old—is born largely out of economic opportunities afforded by patent laws. Drug companies can't typically patent commonly used plants, but they can develop patented, proprietary synthetic drugs, subsequently earning billions in sales.

Dr. Vinod Kumar Gupta, head of India's National Institute of Science Communication and Information Resources, told the BBC in 2005 that of the nearly five thousand patents given out by the U.S. Patent Office on various medical plants up to that time, some eighty per cent were plants of Indian origin.

He and many others call this "bio-piracy" and now they are fighting back. In Delhi in 2005, Ayurvedic practitioners were nearing the end of a massive task: the creation of a thirty-million-page electronic encyclopedia of India's traditional medical knowledge, the first of its kind in the world.

"When we put this encyclopedia in the public domain," said Ajay Dua, a senior bureaucrat in the Commerce Ministry, "no one will be able to claim these medicines or therapies are their inventions. Until now, we have not done the needful to protect our traditional wealth."

Chewing Betel Nut

Do all the nice, older people in the Thai village where I have a home who chew betel feel itchy? Are their sex lives improved?

And what of the millions and millions more in India, Nepal, Sri Lanka, and Burma (where even small boys chew it) and across the rest of Southeast Asia as far as the Philippines? Do they feel their sexual juices begin to boil when they wrap a bit of the areca palm seed in a heart-shaped leaf of the betel pepper along with some other ingredients, stick it between their cheek and their gums and masticate?

These seeds contain alkaloids that have stimulating effects on the body, the mind, and eros. I'm quoting Christian Räatsch in *Plants of Love*, who says the seed is one of the traditional aphrodisiacs of Ayurvedic medicine and is counted among the eight types of pleasure in the Brahmanic tradition, dating back to the *Kama Sutra*. Apparently, there have been no clinical trials; the millennia-long tradition and belief are thought to be "evidence" enough.

Offering betel morsels to guests and visitors is a common courtesy in the Indian sub-continent. Frequently it is served following a meal as a breath-freshener and digestive, and it has been used from ancient times as an aromatic stimulant and anti-flatulent, as well as a household remedy for stomach disorders, headache, constipation, wounds, colds and coughs.

Others say the nut is useful for relieving toothache, stimulating salivation and digestion, preventing perspiration, and treating diarrhea, urinary disorders, smallpox, cholera, and sexually transmitted diseases. Again there is no proof.

The literature says the chew is a mild "narcotic," that the alkaloid in the nut, called *arakene*, is a stimulant or euphoriant, a distant cousin of cocaine. (Very distant, if you ask me, though most scholars agree that it's somewhat addictive.) When I tried it, I felt a tingling sensation in my mouth and lips, accompanied by an elevation of spirit if not anatomy. The taste was bittersweet and the "high" lasted less than an hour.

I watch the women in my village prepare their quid. They slice the unripe, green-hulled nut with the peach-colored interior, using a heavy, hinged metal cutting device, then place a bit on the large green leaf, adding a smear of lime paste (made from coral, limestone or seashells), a chip of fragrant wood, a small twist of cigarette tobacco, folding everything into a neat package. (Cloves, cardamom and other spices may also be added to the mix; local customs vary.)

Over time, the areca nut and lime stain the mouth and saliva red, making those habituated appear to have been hit in the mouth with a tomato and then a plum. That doesn't slow their all-day use of the stuff. Even when they visit the temple, they take their makings with them, sitting in the rear, pounding the ingredients in a mortar with a pestle between blessings and chants, chewing and spitting into tin cans.

I wonder if it makes them horny.

Chapter five
Traditional Chinese Medicine: Better Sex with the Help of the Yellow Emperor

Another contender for "oldest" and "most comprehensive" healthcare system in the world is Traditional Chinese Medicine (TCM). As with Ayurvedic medicine, it goes back some 2,500 to 5,000 years, thus it is rooted in legend—its origins told in fantastical tales—and again as is true in India its numerous preventives and remedies today serve one of the planet's largest populations, while winning a rapidly expanding number of believers worldwide, both inside and outside the Western medical community.

The most important similarity, or parallel, is the quest for "balance" in the body, not in *doshas* as in India but in correcting disharmonies in the *qi* (pronounced "chee"), the vital energy, and imbalances between *yin* and *yang*, the complementary but opposing qualities that represent the natural dualities of the world, such as male/female, day/night, hot/cold, active/passive, et cetera. It's further believed that each organ and body system is related to one of the five elements—wood, fire, earth, metal, and water—and that the body reflects the larger, natural world in this way.

The idea is that if balance is maintained, disease may be prevented, and when it is disturbed, various disciplines of treatment—including herbal remedies, acupressure and acupuncture, dietary and other lifestyle change, therapeutic exercise such as Tai Chi Ch'uan, Kung fu, and other martial arts, and meditation—can restore it. It is a holistic approach to health vastly different from that predominant in the West.

Daniel Reid, an American expatriate who studied Chinese medicine for many years in Taiwan, made this gap clear in *A Handbook of Chinese Healing Herbs* (1995), saying, "While modern Western medicine views disease as a malevolent external invasion by an enemy that must be killed, traditional Chinese medicine sees it more as a matter of 'letting down your guard' and giving entry to the malevolent agents and energies that cause disease. Rather than treating the disease, as modern medicine does, the traditional Chinese physician treats the patient by correcting the critical imbalances in his or her energy system that opened the door to disease in the first place."

Many in the West today brand Chinese medicine unscientific—the more disparaging call it pseudoscience or superstition—and while it's true that many of its claims remain unproven, at least by Western measurement, the system nonetheless is gaining respect and a growing number now treat it as a complementary and alternative medicine, part of the "holistic" or "green medicine" movement that has made such an impact in the past quarter century. By the 1970s, for example, acupuncture was taught at American universities, and meditation and various martial arts were credited with healthful results, as more and more of the herbal remedies simultaneously found their way into the developed world's pharmacopoeias or, at the least, were sold widely as herbal "supplements."

Champions of TCM credit the origins of the medical system to the "Yellow Emperor," Huang Ti, who reigned over a haphazard coalition of tribes around 2700 BC. He also was said to be the first to blend male and female essence (*yin* and *yang*) during intercourse, thereby discovering the secret of eternal immortality, while keeping a harem of more than a thousand women who were his bed buddies frequently, several of them every night. In addition to such stories— reminding me of several I've heard in numerous Asian bars—the Yellow Emperor also left a book called *The Classic of the Plain Girl* that scholars think was first transcribed about the third century BC. This was said to be a record of conversations about sex that he had with three women, which also appear in another text, *The Golden Lotus*. The Yellow Emperor additionally was credited with authoring *The Yellow Emperor's Classic of Internal Medicine*, fount of today's vast TCM pharmacopoeia.

It was also the esteemed emperor who brought so much poetry to sex, offering ten "styles" of intercourse, calling them The Crouching Tiger, The Cricket's Clasp, The Worm That Moves Its Head Back and Forth, The Deer That Lifts Its Horns, The Phoenix Spreads Its Wings, The Climbing Monkey, The Running Hare, The Toad, The Dragonfly, and The Eating Fish.

And wrote: "I have tasted all the medicinal herbs/I have imbibed every medication and potion/And all I need for my health/Is the juice of a young girl."

In the years following publication of such works, TCM developed and spread as far as Europe, its herbs taken away by early traders, missionaries, and diplomats along with the tea and silk. Scholars say TCM peaked during the Ming dynasty (1368–1644 AD), then gradually declined to the status of a folk practice until 1949, when Mao Tse-tung and his People's Republic of China told surviving practitioners to go forth and multiply as a means of making health care available to a population that was then being ignored.

By 2000, at least in China's big cities, the two medicines were being integrated, with less resistance to western diagnostics and treatment than in the West there was resistance to TCM. For example, at a Shanghai cancer hospital, a patient could be seen by a multidisciplinary team and treated concurrently with radiation therapy, Western drugs, and traditional herbal formulas.

When it comes to aphrodisiacs, TCM's variance with Ayurvedic medicine becomes somewhat more pronounced. Concerns about impotency, procreative weakness, frigidity, semen strength, premature ejaculation—and, in fact, the control of ejaculation—were as prevalent, but the scope of ingredients used was quite different. Where in India the therapy was almost totally plant-derived, in China animal ingredients played a significant role. Many of these—including snakes and other reptiles, insects, bear, tiger, rhinoceros, deer, seahorse, and shark—are considered in later chapters of this book. Semen retention, credited to the Yellow Emperor, also gets a subsequent chapter of its own. Now, I want to focus on the herbs, several dozen of the more than two thousand in TCM that are among those prescribed to preserve or restore sexual balance, thus enhancing not only the efficacy but also the enjoyment of sex.

"Like all herbal therapy," wrote Dan Reid in his second classic work, *The Tao of Health, Sex and Longevity* (1988), "aphrodisiacs must be taken over an extended period of time in order to have the desired effects. Since they employ no synthetic chemicals or other artificial ingredients, they must work naturally with the body's circulatory and endocrine systems, and this takes time. Count on two or three months of daily doses for noticeable enhancement of sexual potency to become apparent."

I start with ginseng (*Panax ginseng*), the most famous herb in the entire Chinese pharmacopoeia, what Dan calls "the closest thing to a cure-all that nature has to offer the human species." Native to northeast China, Manchuria, Korea, and Siberia, it used to treat everything from bad gums to memory loss, anemia to impotence. In traditional Japanese medicine, called *kampo*, it is used to control some types of cancer, in Germany it's a remedy for fatigue, in America a panacea for diabetes and hangovers, and just about everywhere it's used to prolong life.

The folk tales that abound say it is the ginseng root's resemblance to the man's body, the tendrils approximating miniature arms, torso, and legs, that put it into the category so prevalent in aphrodisiacs that insists: if it looks like it, it must be good for it. This is a notion that will appear repeatedly in this book and that line of thinking is used, reasonably, by critics as an argument against such so-called substances being worth a damn. Thus, ginseng is placed in a category of aphrodisiac along with tiger penis and rhino horn.

This is unfortunate. Because among all the Chinese plants, ginseng has been taken into western labs more than perhaps any other and established as a substance that can do much that it's been claimed to do for millennia—regulating blood sugar and blood pressure levels along with central nervous system response, relieving fatigue, stimulating the immune system, retarding intoxication when taken prior to drinking, and balancing male and female hormone activity. It's no wonder that ginseng is the most popular Chinese herbal remedy, available worldwide in cola drinks and teas.

However, in order to increase the aphrodisiac effects of

ginseng, the root often is combined with animal ingredients such as tiger bone, dried gecko, toad venom, snake meat, frog concentrate, blister beetle powder, and antler horn.

Ginkgo (*Ginkgo biloba*), believed to be the last surviving plant from the Mesozoic Era (think 150 million years ago, food for dinosaurs), is a tree that grows to some 130 feet (forty meters), native to China and Japan. Most western research has been centered on the fan-shaped leaves, which are thought to have sedative and digestive properties and treat skin and circulation problems, but it is the hard seeds, or kernels, from the large, plum-like fruit that are regarded as sexually enhancing, a food to tonify primordial energy. In Japan, unripe seeds are grilled for this purpose and by publicly consuming the seeds (said Christian Räatsch in *Plants of Love*), "a person can indicate they are not adverse to erotic adventures."

There are many more, including Chinese wild raspberry (*Rubus Coreanus*), whose fruit is used to make jam and leaves are toasted in a hot pan or oven, powdered and taken on an empty stomach with a few ounces of hooch...Chinese wolfberry (*Lycium chinense*), the oval red-orange berries added to so many herbal and reptile wines but also to stews, chicken, and seafood dishes...and Solomon's Seal (*Polygonatum officinale*), sometimes called "Jade Bamboo" for its edible bamboo-like shoots that may also made into an enervating juice, prescribed for impotence. Dan Reid further recommends garlic, pepper, pumpkin seeds (for prostate health), oysters (for the zinc), foxglove, cinnamon, angelica root, and licorice.

Finally we come to the beloved lotus (*Nelumbium nucifera*). To Buddhists, the water lily-like blossom represents the beauty that may emerge from mud, thus it is a symbol of purity, eternal life, and spiritual enlightenment. It also has long been cultivated as a food, for the starchy root and, more commonly, for the raw, ivory colored seeds that are sold in Asian markets as a delicacy.

In TCM, the entire plant is used—the roots for hemostatic and astringent effect, the large, round leaves for heat relief and headache, the stamen as an astringent and remedy for premature ejaculation, the seeds as a mild aphrodisiac. Räatsch says the blossom is a symbol of "the cosmic vagina." Another lovely thought.

Horny Goat Weed & Bald Chicken Tonic

"Long ago, in a remote mountain province of southern China, there lived a goatherd with a very 'horny' herd of goats. His billygoats, it seemed, simply 'couldn't get enough' of their ewes, mounting them and rutting repeatedly in remarkably brief spans of time."

Thus begins a story told by Daniel Reid in his book *The Tao of Sex, Health and Long Life* (1989). When I asked him which, if any, herbal remedies in Traditional Chinese Medicine (TCM) he thought had the most penis punch, it was this one. The story continued:

"The curious goatherd soon noticed a pattern: whenever his billygoats nibbled from a certain patch of weeds, their promiscuous proclivities peaked for hours thereafter. Before long, Chinese herbalists learned what goats had always known: that the plant *Epimedium sagittatum*, a nondescript weed that grows in the wild, is one of the most potent male aphrodisiacs on earth. Logically, they named the new medicinal herb *Yin-Yang-huo*—'Horny Goat Weed'."

Dan lived in Asia for many years (mainly in Taiwan and Thailand), studying from the original ancient texts, and in his later book, *A Handbook of Chinese Healing Herbs*, he suggested three ways to prepare the leaves of the plant for consumption. The first was by decoction, a process that called for boiling and then simmering the leaves in water, then drinking the liquid warm between meals on an empty stomach.

The leaves could also be dried and powdered, then taken by the spoonful and chased with a glass of wine or saké, or in a tea or in capsule form. Powdered herbs act more slowly and "gently" than decoctions, he said, and the effect is less intense and lasts longer.

The third method calls for steeping the herbs in strong distilled spirits for three months to a year. This, he said, was the most effective way.

Horny Goat Weed was not the only Chinese herb named for a non-human species. What is called the Bald Chicken Tonic is a potion reputed to have helped an ancient Chinese gentleman, the prefect of Shu, Lu Ta-ching, sire three sons after he was seventy. A teaspoon of the stuff taken with wine once a day for sixty days purportedly will enable a man to fornicate up to forty women a day. The way the story goes, Lu Ta-ching so wore out one of his partners, what remained of the tonic was thrown into the courtyard, where it was consumed by a rooster. Thus energized, the cock jumped on a nearby chicken and screwed it nonstop for a number of days, pecking the hen's head until it was bald.

Should all of this sound like something from a Chinese comic strip, it should be noted that Horny Goat Weed was one of the twenty most popular traditional Chinese medicines sold in the U.S. in 2004.

Chapter six
Jammin' with Jamu

A woman of about fifty arrived outside two side-by-side massage brothels in Jakarta's Chinatown. Strapped to her back was a woven basket packed with liter-sized bottles of colored liquid, a load that weighed at least twenty kilograms (forty-four pounds) when she began her morning rounds. She also had with her some fresh duck eggs and a plastic bag full of commercially packaged herbs. She set the basket down outside one of the doors and poked her head inside. She was recognized and an order was placed.

The woman selected one of the eggs and neatly removed one end with a small knife, carefully pouring the albumen into the gutter, leaving the yolk. She then filled the shell almost to the top with an orange liquid, added a splash of something between purple and black, then carried it through the brothel door.

The woman was one of the thousands of *jamu gendong*, the sidewalk vendors of medicinal herbs who twice a day patroled city streets in Indonesia, selling powders and drinks with which to begin the day or night. The use of Javanese herbs in a curative or health-giving capacity was centuries old and although many were aimed at preventing or treating disease or toning the skin cosmetically, the most popular were those believed to enhance sexual performance. Chinatown was Jakarta's "red light district," so it was here where many of the vendors joined noodle sellers in the morning and again at dusk on the busy streets.

With a friend who spoke Bahasa Indonesia, as the sun sank into Jakarta's smog, I strolled again along one of the Chinatown thoroughfares. Here, every couple of blocks, near the brothels and discos and music lounges and short-time hotels, men took over the *jamu* trade, positioning carts adjacent to worn tables and benches. A large banner hung from the awning overhead hid the stand from pedestrian and vehicular passersby. On the cart we approached was a glass case where the packaged *jamu lake-lake* (man's medicine) was displayed. Next to the glass case were bottles of honey with ginger, a small basket of duck eggs and limes.

Nearby at another table two Indonesian men sat, hunkered over their glasses of herbal brew, getting a big kick out of seeing two white faces in what normally was a locals only environment.

"They're getting a giggle out of this," my friend said.

"Yeah, and they'd probably fall off the bench if we actually drank any of this stuff."

One of the two young boys in charge of the stall explained that his family had been selling *jamu* at this spot for twenty years. He said we could either have a glass of the pre-blended liquid on the spot or buy some of the powdered *jamu lake-lake* to take home. Most of the packages featured idealized drawings of muscle men or Bima, one of the Hindu gods portrayed in *Ramayana*, the epic tale that dated back millennia and came to Indonesia from India. We were told the powders were to be mixed with warm water and a generous dollop of honey, the latter presumably to kill the ingredients' bitter taste.

Jamu is like—and not like—the herbal pharmacopoeias of India, China, and the Himalayas. All rely on indigenous plants as a treatment for illness, but mainly as a means of toning and balancing the body and thereby *preventing* disease. As was true with the other systems, it was believed that the herbal help worked best when part of a larger regime; in Indonesia, this encompassed spiritual, religious, mystical, magical and herbal elements, as well as a form of massage. Plus: a balancing of heat and cold, thus hot medicine cured a cold illness and cold medicine was recommended for a hot ailment, and when *jamu* was given to treat a problem in one part of the body the effect on the rest of the body was to be considered as well. Also, any one "prescription" could include more than a dozen ingredients. And none promised instant results. The herbal potions, powders, and pills were suggested for long-term rather than quick effect. So daily use was required for a period of several months before response should fairly be judged.

A big difference was the role of alcohol. In China and India, the herbs could be mixed with rice wine or other alcoholic beverages, and, in fact, were often recommended. In Indonesia, *jamu* was *never* mixed with alcohol, as it was believed it would neutralize the herbs' effectiveness. Only water was used.

No one knows how old *jamu* is. The earliest surviving manuscript, *Serat Centhini*, dates back only to the eighteenth century, when three men were commissioned by the ruler of the central Javanese kingdom of Surakarta to conduct a general study of all spiritual, material, scientific, and religious knowledge (and not just *jamu*). Sixteen volumes were produced, much of it resembling a series of fairy tales, including one that said a poorly endowed Javanese man searched far and wide before discovering a mushroom that not only made his penis strong, but increased its circumference and length, thus saving his marriage.

Other manuscripts, housed today in a library in Solo, one of the major cities in Java, encompass some five thousand texts written on seven hundred thousand pieces of paper, which are bound into approximately two thousand volumes. The subject matter is wide, but many have sections devoted to "pharmacy, prescriptions and recipes."

So pervasive was the belief in *jamu*, only a few decades ago, as part of a marriage trousseau, brides were customarily given square- or pyramid-shaped boxes with drawers filled with medicinal herbs designed to make the marriage a successful one.

In *Jamu: The Ancient Indonesian Art of Herbal Healing* (2001), the author, Susan-Jane Beers, gives what seems a simplistic yet plausible explanation why so many so-called aphrodisiacs are a key part of *jamu*. "Why did appearance and sexual attraction become an obsession in Indonesia, an Islamic country where traditional values are extremely strong?" she asked. "The answer may be in the position that Indonesian men hold in the family unit—one that can assume a quasi-godlike status. This attitude is reinforced by Islamic law, a law that allows men to acquire up to four wives provided they can support them adequately." Sexually as well as financially.

Thus in modern Indonesia, as in ancient India and China,

there were multiple partners to satisfy, so any little help from the garden or nearby rain forest was much appreciated. Also, Beers said, "in the past, Islam made it relatively easy for men to obtain a divorce and the unlucky wives would be left without a breadwinner, usually with young families to support." Given these circumstances, she wrote, it was no wonder a wife took efforts to hold her husband's attention.

"Indonesian custom dictates that female health and beauty are inextricably bound up with a woman's role as wife and mother, which means sex is a key element in the equation," Beers explained. "Naturally, *jamu* reflects these beliefs and is biased in favor of good health, beauty, marital harmony, sex and large families. Staying attractive was (and often still is) of economic as well as social importance."

In a "cure" suggested following the birth of a child, the woman took a hot bath as the *jamu* masseuse prepared charcoal in a kind of brazier. The woman then stood over the burning charcoal to warm her body and tighten the vaginal muscles. Next came a herbal oil body massage to restore body tone. A poultice of cajput oil, juice of a thin-skinned lime and *kapur sirih*—a mixture of lime powder and betel leaves—was mixed with *tapel* powder to form a paste, which was applied to the stomach. According to Susan-Jane Beers, this dispelled any blood remaining in the womb, firmed the muscles and contracted the stomach, helping mom regain her figure.

As evident here and as was also true in India and China, concoctions were often complex, a *jamu* formula consisting of as many as forty or more ingredients. (Some of these were secondary, inactive items, used to disguise the medicine's bitterness or to mask offensive odors.) Until the 1980s, virtually all the *jamu* was made at home by those who sold them.

With ingredients purchased from collectors who went into the forests or from wholesale markets, the *jamu gendong* were up long before dawn to chop and mix and stir, filling heavy bottles made especially for the trade and handed down for generations, stoppering them with folds of banana leaf. There was a great deal of secrecy attached to this, no one *jamu* maker willing to divulge his or her formulas, the ingredients and their quantities often differing substantially, although the names given the blends did not.

All of this led to difficulties in testing such remedies clinically. So as Indonesian doctors and pharmacists—and businesses seeing commercial opportunity—wanted a more scientific approach to the manufacture and prescription of *jamu*, the Ministry of Health ruled in the 1990s that all commercial producers had to reduce formulas for curing to five essential ingredients. The government also required clinical trials for both medical drugs and traditional medicine to be conducted to satisfy the same costly criteria as required in the West, a problem for *jamu* makers who realized small profit because prices charged were low. The four packets of powdered *jamu* I bought from the night street vendor together came to less than $2.50. And I was probably paying the *bule* (foreigner) price.

I had missed the early morning rounds of the *jamu gendong*, the first of the day's heavy trafficking. This was when the vendors, almost all of them women, went from door to door with their baskets to offer cosmetic and medicinal drinks by the glass to housewives and deliver special orders, usually wrapped in a banana leaf. My interest was in the evening trade, when men had finished work and now anticipated a few hours of *jamu*, women, and song. Where the morning vendors were almost exclusively women, now the majority were men, selling their powders and potions in the greatest number in the "red light" neighborhoods.

Even more were sold, mainly in loose powder or capsule form, in commercial pharmacies fed not by *jamu gendong* but by a crowd of professional manufacturers. Susan-Jane Beers reported, "By the 1980s, a few medium sized *jamu* producers had grown sufficiently to introduce large-scale, modern production methods. Ten years later, Indonesia's *jamu* industry comprised around five hundred companies, including twenty major players."

Thus in 2006 in Indonesia, I could watch *jamu* commercials on television and I was able to find on a shelf alongside brand name western medicines such *jamu* as Pasak Bumi (whose bitter bark was considered the most powerful male aphrodisiac), Sehat Pria (described as a "prophylactic herbal tea for men only" by one manufacturer, as an "*aprodisiak* and *anti impotensi*" by another), Kuku Bima (with ginseng and seahorse added), and a wide range of other blends, as well as a leaf with the local name of *down seri* that evidently kept women's vaginas dry and odor free while strengthening the musculature.

Still, *jamu* makers had not yet found much of a foreign market. Without "scientific proof," thousands of years of use on the street in a country on the other side of the world meant little to the ED thousands, even hundreds of miles away. Still, with expanded interest in traditional medicines and a holistic approach to well-being growing worldwide, a few countries were showing serious interest. By the late 1990s, the Netherlands, onetime colonial rulers of Indonesia, allowed imports of *jamu* in quantity…and perhaps it was no coincidence that Anita Roddick spent many years researching health and beauty products in Indonesia (as well as in

Nepal) before opening her chain of stores called Body Shop.

Jamu was also being sold on the Internet. One site I came across that offered *jamu* to "spice up your sex live," started its page with a bit of enticing gibberish: "*jamu* Indonesia sex herb Viagra tight vagina premature *ejaculatin kuda* better sex *jamu* aphrodisiac impotence beautiful *impotentie erektie* gay lesbian *bali sanrego.*"

How could anyone resist?

Chapter seven
The Spices of Life

If there were no Maluku, the Indonesian province that includes the tiny volcanic islands of Ambon, Ternate, and Banda, also known as the "Spice Islands," there might not have been an America.

This is an absurd statement, but it isn't without some foundation in fact. When Columbus set forth under royal Spanish patronage at the end of the fifteenth century to find an easy passage to what then were called the Moluccas, he was convinced the islands lay at the far side of the Atlantic Ocean. Columbus encountered the Caribbean and the Americas instead.

Thus distracted, other Europeans got to Indonesia first, starting with the Portuguese in 1514, through force gaining a monopoly they held for almost a hundred years. At the time, the Moluccas—northeast of Timor and west of Irian Jaya— were the only source of clove, nutmeg, and mace in economically feasible quantity. Small amounts had reached Europe as early as the twelfth century, finding favor among those

wealthy enough to afford them, and now the market exploded. Seeing Portuguese spice merchants grow rich, the Dutch
wrested control in 1609, and they were followed a year later
in small number by the English.

The islanders were not happy about the prices paid by the
Dutch and began selling to the English. The Dutch responded by imposing the death penalty on anyone possessing nutmeg, mace, or cloves without their authorization and in a fif-
teen-year period (1621–1636), Japanese mercenaries working for the Dutch East Indies Company tortured, quartered,
and beheaded Bandanese leaders, impaling their heads on
bamboo poles for public display, then destroyed the villages
and killed their inhabitants until the population had been
reduced from fifteen thousand to less than a thousand.

The Dutch then added herbicide to genocide, burning all
the nutmeg trees on Banda, an act that limited production
and thus kept prices high, and at the same time put all surviving groves in the shadow of Dutch forts on other islands.
This permitted the Dutch to increase the price of nutmeg
from what they paid in the Moluccas to what was charged
on the open market in Amsterdam by more than a thousand
per cent.

As Richard Bangs and Christian Kallen noted in their
book *Islands of Fire, Islands of Spice* (1988), there remained
"the nagging matter" of the English, whose interest in the
islands seemed most threatening to the Dutch quest for
complete monopoly. Rather than go to war, the Dutch
offered the English a deal: if England would go away, they'd
give the Brits their only North American possession, a small
city they considered unimportant called New Amsterdam, on
an island called Manhattan. Such are the vagaries of history.

After a hundred and fifty years, the Dutch East Indies
Company went bankrupt, and the English returned briefly,

but following the Napoleonic Wars in Europe in the early nineteenth century, control was restored to the Dutch. The mystique of the Spice Islands finally died when France successfully smuggled seeds and plants to Mauritius, Britain doing the same to establish plantations in Penang, Sri Lanka, Sumatra, Singapore, and Grenada, thus making spices a more commonplace and affordable commodity.

"For centuries nutmeg was used to flavor and preserve foods, binding together diverse tastes into a coherent whole," wrote Nigel Simmonds in *Banda: A Journey Through Indonesia's Fabled Isles of Fire and Spice* (1997). "Its bitter agent was used to round out the flavor of meat, enhancing both sweet and savory. It was used as a medicine to help bronchial disorders, rheumatism, and digestion. Later, it became a cure-all, an aphrodisiac and a mark of civility…the seventeenth century wonder drug, more expensive than silver, more sought after than money, more coveted than gold."

The word "nutmeg" is misleading, because it is not a true nut, but a single seed found in the apricot-sized fruit of a tree that grows to about sixty feet (eighteen meters). The dark brown seed is wrapped in a fibrous and somewhat lacy, vermillion covering that, when dried, is known as mace, making the species unique in producing two distinct spices from one tree. The seeds are dried on shallow trays of open basketwork and heated over a slow fire for up to three months. The blackened shell is then broken and the nutmeg, now rattling inside, is removed for processing and marketing. Stored in an airtight container, they will keep indefinitely, but once grated or crushed, the volatile oils and accompanying fragrance quickly dissipate.

The bulk of the product is now grown in Grenada in the Caribbean. Nutmeg oil, extracted from the seed, leaves, and bark, is used to add taste to carbonated soft drinks and other foods, and in the production of perfumes. In many Western countries it is sprinkled atop frothy alcoholic drinks such as eggnog, in Britain added to rice puddings, egg custards, and other milk dishes. In India, it appears in Moghul dishes, in France in patés, terrines and sausages, in Italy with veal and sauces for pasta. In Asia, it is still considered a strong medicine, as a gargle, a purgative, or a cure for diarrhea.

Its reputation as an aphrodisiac is mixed, but of all the many spices that appear on the long shelf of dictionaries and encyclopedias and texts on the subject, it is one of the most frequently praised. More importance than is surely due may be attributed to the tree's own botanical character. Both male and female trees occur and one male can fertilize up to a dozen female trees, prompting one writer to call it "the *passia* of tropical flora"—for the umpteenth time, giving men an excuse to say, "If nature can do that, if I consume that part of nature, I can do it, too." There is also what may be an apocryphal tale told about the French painter Henri de Toulouse-Lautrec, who was reputed to carry a small grater and nutmeg cloves in order to flavor his port in Parisian brothels, and though he was hardly what today is called a "hunk"—he was, in fact, a dwarf—it's claimed the ladies all loved him for his sexual potency.

The most convincing "proof" came when scientists took two of nutmeg's essential oils, *isosafrole* and *myristicine*, and used their chemistry as blueprints for the drugs known as MDA and MDMA. The former, first synthesized in Germany in 1910, has been called the "drug of truth" and "speed for lovers." It is believed to enhance tactile sensitivity, feelings of intimacy, and the ability to communicate with a sexual partner. MDMA, also thought to help lovers open up to each other psychologically and provide intense physical pleasure, is better known as Ecstasy and has been the drug of choice for

Asia's late night disco crowd for more than a decade, from Taipei to Jakarta to Bangkok to Mumbai. (See "Better Loving, Through Chemistry," page 173.) In the original, or nutmeg form, a hallucinogenic effect accompanies the ingestion of at least two whole nutmegs, freshly grated, consumed dregs and all in a tea or other potable.

The list of spices credited with aphrodisiacal powers is not short, but no list of aphrodisiacal plants ever is. Somewhere in the world at some time, celery, carrot, banana, and asparagus (what do they look like, after all?), potato, apple, avocado, pomegranate, durian, wheat, garlic, pineapple, lotus, the roots of chervil and fern, mustard, coconut, dates, walnuts, almonds, radish, and many more garden crops have been credited with such power.

Besides nutmeg, the list of spices includes another dozen plants, most of them if not indigenous to Asia, found in Asia now and popular in various Asian cuisines as well as in potion and pill. Rarely is one of them taken alone, rather they are added to other herbs and foods for what the consumer hopes will add a little something besides improved taste.

Next on my Aphrodisiac Hit Parade is an item frequently thought of as a spice, but it, too, is not. *Allium sativum*, or **garlic**, is the most powerfully flavored member of the onion family and is, in fact, a bulb or sort of root. Indigenous to Central Asia, it is now cultivated over the entire earth and is an indispensable ingredient to many dishes and cuisines.

In *Bruce Cost's Asian Ingredients: Buying and Cooking the Staple Foods of China, Japan and Southeast Asia* (1988), an excellent introduction to as well as the close-to-final word on the subject (for my money), the author said Asians consumed "the most garlic per capita on earth, measurably more than the people of the Mediterranean. Korea is first in the world, although the Chinese in the far north consume about as much as the Koreans; Thailand is second; and the countries that surround Thailand—Laos, Cambodia, and Vietnam—would put the Italians and Greeks to shame." I'm sure it's still true.

It's sure true in my home, where my Khmer-Thai wife may begin the day frying pounded garlic and chili peppers in a wok with oil. All the windows are open, the exhaust fan over the stove is turned on, and incense is burning nearby, yet still the effect is, for a foreigner like me, overpowering. If I'm in the next room working at the computer, Lamyai will kindly close the door. But if I'm near the stove, it's like the breath is being sucked from my lungs and I cough, I weep. The same thing happens on the street when vendors cook their most popular condiments for seasoning the day's stir-fries. I walk by and it's as if I've entered an asthma-like Twilight Zone.

I love it.

Garlic—a bulb like its cousin the onion that is actually odor-free until it is sliced or crushed—is a food rich in minerals and offering many medicinal qualities for which the bulb is famed, including antibacterial, antifungal, and anti-thrombotic, the latter referring to its keeping the blood from clotting. This is one of those plants that really does seem to work medical miracles.

Some say it works as an aphrodisiac, too. In *Plants of Joy*, Christian Räatsch said, "Its aphrodisiac usefulness was known to the ancient Egyptians. The Romans consecrated it to Ceres, the Goddess of Fertility, and made a love drink from pressed garlic juice and coriander. Many old books on herbs state that garlic leads to lascivious behavior. It is also claimed that garlic can heal impotency brought about by witchcraft. It is often said that meals heavy in garlic have erotic effects." It all sounds empirical rather than clinical to me, so who knows. But you can't help liking the author's enthusiasm.

Cinnamon, the dried bark of *Cinnamomum verum*, a tree indigenous to Sri Lanka, is next. This spice drew attention of Roman traders as early as the sixth century BC and has been, along with tea, one of Sri Lanka's most profitable agricultural crops.

Cinnamon is believed to be one of the oldest spices—it's mentioned in Sanskrit texts—and it was in ancient times used to flavor wine. In the Middle Ages, it was put in stews, soups, custards, and poultry fricassees, and today is used in compotes and desserts and to add a spicy flavor to mulled wine. In modern Asia its applications are more numerous and it's routinely added to a multitude of dishes.

While the bark is what appears in stick or powdered form in shops and restaurants, the leaves and branches are used for distilling a thick, pungent oil in the perfume industry and as a remedy against colds. As all parts of the tree, which grows to about thirty or so feet (ten meters), exude the aroma, when standing near a cinnamon, be prepared to be transported, as the scent is somewhat exciting. Cinnamon oil may also be rubbed on the genitals for erotic stimulation or, so it's said.

The fifth all-time, I-want-it spice for me is good old **black** pepper, *Piper nigrum*, first harvested in India, introduced to Java as early at 100 BC by Hindus who created kingdoms there, spread to China a hundred or so years later, and to Japan in the eighth century (where it hasn't been all that accepted as a common spice). By the Middle Ages, pepper assumed great importance in Europe where it was cherished by the rich as a seasoning. In Antwerp in the mid sixteenth century, quoting *The Oxford Companion to Food (1999)*, "the price of pepper served as a barometer for European business in general."

The most popular and most widespread spice in the world today, pepper grows on a climbing vine that may stretch for fifty feet (fifteen meters) and the smaller-than-pea-sized fruit hangs from stems like bunches of grapes. It blooms year-round and thus is continuously ripening. Black and white pepper are widely available, their differences based on how they were processed—the black sold dried and of the two, offering the most bite, the white having had its outer husk removed in salt water, providing a somewhat weaker kick.

It's a staple in China, where the "hot" in Hot and Sour Soup is the white peppercorn. In Vietnam, Thailand, and Indonesia, black peppercorns are ground with other spices and fresh herbs to make curry pastes, or the ground pepper is sprinkled over dishes as is done in Western cooking.

Here's Räatsch again: "Both Asian and European folk medicinal traditions consider pepper a good aphrodisiac. It contains an alkaloid (*piperline*) that irritates the mucous membranes. Cubeb pepper (*Piper cubeba*), which is closely related, grows in Indonesia. Also ingested as an aphrodisiac, cubeb contains a substance that stimulates the sex drive." Again there is no clinical backup. But as anyone who has sprinkled a little too much pepper on a dish knows, the result can be incendiary.

The last is cardamom, the fruit of a perennial herb, *Elettaria cardamomum*, the world's third most costly spice, after saffron and vanilla. (So how can all those vanilla ice cream cones be so cheap? It ain't real vanilla.) Indigenous to South India and Sri Lanka and traded for a thousand years, today it is grown mainly in India, Guatemala, Sri Lanka, and Tanzania, with Papua New Guinea, China, and Sumatra following at some distance behind.

The fruits are picked before they are ripe and dried until

they become hard and green in color. The seeds inside the fruit, turning from white to black as it ripens, are what produce the pleasant aroma and slightly pungent flavor. Cardamom is used much more in Asia than in Europe, save for Scandinavia where it's added to mulled wines, stewed fruits, and flans. Its most common use is in India, where it flavors rice, cakes, omelets, meat and noodle dishes, and beverages such as tea, coffee, and *bhang*, the latter both a hallucinogenic and an aphrodisiac (see "Medical Marijuana" page 95). Cardamom, like nutmeg and so many other spices, loses a lot of its power in the processing and the time it takes to reach Asian supermarket shelves.

Christian Räatsch, whose text is hard to forget, suggests a "love drink" made by mixing a heaping teaspoon of ground coffee with the same amount of ground cardamom, brewing in the usual way. Add milk and sugar or honey to taste and, Räatsch promises, "The effects are quickly noticeable."

I tried it and Christian Räatsch was correct. The smell of coffee and cardamom didn't go away for several days.

Chapter eight
Tempest in a C-Cup & Other Arousing Tales

On February 25, 2005, a Thai pop star, Prisna "Pookie" Praisaeng (already regarded as a controversial figure for having a child out of wedlock and bragging about it) and three other models were fined for staging a public demonstration of a breast-firming cream that had the models posing topless before a pack of enthusiastic Bangkok journalists as they massaged the product into their breasts.

The models were paid ($75 each) to pose for fifteen minutes and Pookie was identified as an executive of the company. The models were fined about the equivalent of $6 apiece for indecent exposure, Pookie was fined the same amount for hiring them, and a few days later the product, St Herb Nano Breast Cream, was temporarily pulled from store shelves by Thailand's Food and Drug Administration for improper labeling.

The interesting thing about this stunt was not its brazen nature—this was Thailand, after all—but there seemed to be some possibility that the main ingredient in the cream had some value. At least it had one champion, Dr. Wichai Cherdshewasart of Chulalongkorn University's Faculty of Science, who said the native herbal plant known as *kwao krua* had potential not only as an effective breast-enhancer, but also in fighting ageing and cancer and, depending on the species of this root of a creeper plant found in the jungles of northern Thailand, Burma, and Laos, as a remedy for erectile dysfunction.

It was five years earlier, in 1999, when Dr. Wichai first made himself known to the press, hailing red *kwao krua* (*Butea superba*) as a herbal "Thai Viagra". Unlike Viagra, Dr. Wichai said his herbal remedy had to be consumed for three to four days before taking effect and he got Thailand's FDA to approve his product as a "traditional Thai medicine."

The years passed as numerous products based on *kwao krua* were approved by the Thai FDA and went onto the marketplace. Then in 2004 it was learned that Japan had hijacked Thailand by obtaining patents in the U.S. for the plant two years earlier, in 2002. Once Thailand's largest market for *kwao krua*, the Japanese had obtained some seeds and started growing it themselves.

There were calls to invalidate the U.S. patents, just as there would be similar cries to protect Thailand's beloved jasmine rice, which had been showing up in Cambodia, and the funny little three-wheeled taxi called a *tuk-tuk* that was appearing in a modified form on European streets. Alas, it was too late. For jasmine rice, for *tuk-tuks*, and for Pookie's make-em-bigger cream.

The lesson here is that anything related to sex seems to win easy attention in the media, thus hardly a day goes by without our being tossed another tidbit, designed to tempt and titillate. So it is with aphrodisiacs, which seem to pop up everywhere in Asia as the Arousing Herb of the Month.

Thailand's kwao krua was just one.

In Malaysia, it was *tongkat ali*, also known (conveniently) as Longjack for its botanical name *Eurycoma longifolia jack*. In Vietnam, it was called *cay ba binh* (the plant that cures a hundred ills), in Indonesia, *pasak bumi*. In 2005 in the Southeast Asian press, few plants received so much attention, often being ranked along with African *yohimbe* and Siberian ginseng as the stuff that really worked, not only in the bedroom but also on the athletic field in building energy, stamina, blood circulation, and muscle mass. Mother Nature's own steroid, some called it. Others pointed proudly to a study by the School of Pharmaceutical Science at Universiti Sains Malaysia that claimed when impotent rats were given doses of the root extract for twelve weeks, the rats "seemed to have a high level of ejaculation." (Rats? As calmly as I could, I reminded myself that this was the way many miracle drugs were tested.)

Traditionally, the entire plant, which may grow to thirty feet (ten meters) and also is found in Indonesia, Thailand, Burma, and Vietnam, can be used for medicinal purposes, but it is the root that was consumed most often. Because of its bitter taste, the boiled root extract usually was dried and powdered and sold in capsule form. As was the case with so many other so-called aphrodisiacs it was not hailed as a quick pick-me-up, but something to be taken long-term before any results were to be expected, some manufacturers spiking the capsules with *sildenafil nitrate* to hurry the process along.

Another media favorite, what might be termed a "perennial," was the fruit of the genus *Capsicum frutescens*. This is the world-famous chili pepper, a bushy plant that thrives in tropical climates just about everywhere and is believed to have made the trip from its native Latin America to Asia in the holds of Portuguese trading ships. Today it's difficult to think of many Asian cuisines without it, especially those of Thailand and India.

Chilis are "hot" because they contain *capsaicin*. This is an irritant alkaloid found mainly in the interior tissue to which the seeds adhere. (So if you want what the Thais call *phet nit noi*, or "little heat," instead of *phet mak mak*, or "six alarm fire," gut and scrape the insides of the little buggers before adding them to a recipe. Another rule of thumb is: the smaller the chilis, the hotter the fire.) According to the guys in Oxford, "*Capsaicin* has at least five separate chemical components; three give immediate sensation in the throat and at the back of the palate, the other two a slower, longer-lasting, and less fierce hotness on the tongue and mid-palate." Cooks use chili for flavor, not merely for hotness and in Asia it is famous for its use in salads, soups, curries, and, in dried and powdered form, as an everyday condiment. Synthetic *capsaicin* is used in anti-mugger sprays.

It's also used to encourage—or, more accurately, enhance—sex. Because the oil found in the flesh is an irritant, we are warned to avoid contact with the eyes or any sensitive skin. Some find this not a danger but an attribute. Yes, keep it away from the eyes, but other sensitive flesh might enjoy it when applied. Its more commonplace mode of consumption in food may cause the face to flush, increase body temperature and blood pressure, thus it is not just an irritant but also a powerful stimulant.

The Oxford Encyclopedia points out that "the discomfort in the mouth causes the brain to produce endorphins, natural opiates that give pleasure." This could mean that those who begin eating chili peppers from a young age—as is ordinary throughout much of South and Southeast Asia—are, in fact, "mildly" addicted, missing it enormously when deprived of it.

I cannot think about chilis without recalling an experience I had in one of the more notorious neighborhoods in Bangkok back when I was unmarried and new to Thailand, thus in a state of testosterone overdrive. When I entered the bar in mid-afternoon, I was the only customer and the girls who worked there were finishing lunch. I ordered a beer and after a while I was approached by a young woman who had just finished a bowl of *som tam*, the fiery green papaya salad made with as many hot chili peppers as the consumer can possibly survive. As I drank my beer, she went to work and the residual heat that the peppers had left behind in her mouth was passed along to me.

It was much later when I learned that Traditional Chinese Medicine employed pepper-laced liniments to achieve warming effects in external applications. "Cayenne plasters are excellent analgesics that help with circulation," said David Molony, executive director of the American Association of Oriental Medicine. "You can throw some cayenne in your socks or shoes to make your feet feel warmer, too." And maybe into your underwear, as well, I thought.

By far the most unusual media darling of recent years hit the headlines in the warming days of spring every year in western Nepal when poor farmers and villagers walked for up to fifteen days to the Dolpo region in the Himalayan foothills. In Dolpo itself, government offices were deserted and the schools went unattended, as even the youngest children joined the annual pilgrimage.

Between the middle of May and the end of June, more than thirty thousand people trekked into one of the poorest and least developed regions of one of the most impoverished countries in the world to spend weeks on their knees, collecting a half-caterpillar and half-mushroom called a *yarchagumba*, Tibetan for "herb of life." Media called it the "Love Bug."

As the cold winter snows receded ahead of the rainy season, spores of the *Cordyceps sinesis* mushroom attacked a burrowing moth larva found just beneath the earth's surface, sinking its roots into the caterpillar's brain, eventually killing it before emerging from the soil. It was the tiny fused fungus and larva that all those school children, bureaucrats, and trekkers were looking for, believing stories about yaks that ate the half plant/half bug and "frolicked with great energy and passion" (quoting an enthusiastic Internet site)—thus adding one more tall tale to the folklore that said if it made an animal frisky, so, too, it would make me.

To the Nepalese, it was a goldmine. A picker who found ten *yarchagumba* a day could earn about $5 from local traders, a small fortune in a country where the majority of the population were subsistence farmers operating outside the cash economy.

The market for the critter was, and still is, mainly in China (especially in what used to be called Tibet), South Korea, and Japan, where the creatures sold for as much as $2,800 per kilogram. (Because of their small size and insignificant weight, it took about 3,500 *yarchagumba* to make up a kilogram.) Powdered and served in a tonic or soup, or used to stuff a duck which was then boiled, it was thought that the *yarchagumba* was not only an aphrodisiac, but also a sort of panacea: strongly antioxidant, antiviral, antibacterial, anticancer, and it was believed to moderate blood pressure and blood sugar, reduce cholesterol, and protect and tone the liver, kidney, heart, and nervous system. It was also taken for shortness of breath, asthma, soreness of loins and knees, dizziness, and tinnitus.

Clinical tests didn't prove any of this, yet the critter had some impressive champions. One of the most prized herbs in Chinese medicine, it nonetheless was substantially unknown outside China until in 1992 when that country's Olympic women's track team athletes broke multiple world records and attributed their success in part to the "Love Bug" they took as an herbal supplement.

Another kicker to the story came in 2004, when it was learned that it was being used to finance a war. That was when Major Jeitendra Karki, the Royal Nepalese army officer responsible for the district of Dolpo, said the Maoists rebels who controlled the area made between $700,000 and $900,000 taxing the trade, using that cash to buy weapons and other supplies. Collectors paid the Maoists a fee to enter the area, another on the way out depending on how many of the creatures they found. The middlemen to whom they sold their find, who then wholesaled them in Tibet and elsewhere, were also taxed.

In the 1960s, there was a slogan put forward to protest the American war in Vietnam: Make Love, Not War. Now it was possible to do both.

Chapter nine
"Medical Marijuana"

"Why do you cook with *ganja*?" I asked a friend who was a cook with her own restaurant a couple of hours outside Bangkok, a small place that catered to the local trade.

"I don't know."

"Come on. Do you do it to get your customers high? Does it taste good? Is it medicine? What?"

"They know *ganja*," she finally said. "Smoke *ganja*, they come eat soup with me. They not say nothing. They not big mouth. They come for beep soup, curry. Li' dat."

She said it was the first thing she did in the morning before opening the restaurant. She took a handful of chopped, sun-dried chili peppers and fried them in a pan without oil with some dried and crumbled marijuana flowers and leaves, removing everything from the fire when she saw the first sign of smoke. That meant the *tetrahydrocannabinol*, or THC, had been activated in the *ganja*. She then pounded the two herbs in a mortar, stored the result in a jar beside the stove, and on request from her regular customers, added the blend to the curries and beep soup.

Or, she said, she combined small amounts (she pinches the end of her little finger) of galangal, lemongrass, ginger, garlic, red chilis, and *ganja*—fresh, not dried—pounding them into a paste, then added the uncooked sticky mixture to whatever was ordered from her menu.

Less frequently, she said, she put the marijuana and other ingredients into a cheesecloth bag, boiled it in water, and then used the liquid as a soup stock, adding noodles, meat, vegetables and so on.

"With everything, cook!" she exclaimed.

"So," I repeated, "why do you cook with *ganja*?"

She smiled and said, "Make man strong. Oh, boy."

Experts who have studied marijuana—and many, many have—insist that there is nothing in it that activates anything connected to the libido or the sexual organs. Some say it acts in reverse, distracting users with hallucinations and eating binges and the like. In 1972, the U.S. National Commission on Marijuana and Drugs expressed doubt that cannabis directly stimulated sexual feelings…echoing the conclusion reached almost eighty years before when a similar commission in India studied the plant. In addition, the practitioners of traditional systems of medicines (TSM) in India who prescribed *ganja* for thousands of years, admitted it could cause mental confusion, drowsiness, and excessive garrulousness, three states of mind that may not lead rapidly to a really terrific roll in the hay. Even what I consider the best book ever written about marijuana, *Cannabis: A History* by Martin Booth (2003), a book so wonderfully exhaustive in its research that *The Guardian* in its review said another serious look at the notorious *Cannabis sativa* would not be needed for a hundred years, stated flatly that "The long-held belief that cannabis is an aphrodisiac has been discounted. Any romantic inclination felt whilst intoxicated is due to the temporary suspension of an individual's natural reticence rather than a chemical effect upon hormones or whatever else might control libido."

A left-handed compliment, if I ever heard one. That "temporary suspension of an individual's natural reticence" has also been attributed to alcohol. (About which, more soon.) When inhibitions are lowered and perhaps erased, fantasies are sometimes made real.

Generally speaking, there are four areas that have been noticed and explored. The first is the joy of *ganja*. A member of the hemp family that grows freely just about everywhere except in the Arctic and in Antarctica, it is the most widely used recreational "drug" in the world. Without a doubt, the Number One reason for smoking or ingesting it is to get what the consumer calls "high." On this point, there is no disagreement. Most people say it reduces anxiety and relaxes the user while intensifying experience of the senses, especially sound, taste, and touch. Back in the 1960s and 1970s when I was one of its champions—and was arrested for growing it—we called it "Psychedelic, man!" Even the ancient Chinese agreed, Taoists using it as a hallucinogen by adding it to other ingredients in incense burners.

The second focus is more pragmatic. That is to say, commercial. Hemp is one of the oldest and one of history's most important fiber and oilseed plants and likely was an important trade item from a very early date. Close to where it's believed to have originated untold millennia ago, in north and northeast China, painted pottery from the Neolithic Yang-shao culture (c. 4200–3200 BC) indicates the presence of cultivated hemp, when it was, as now in some parts of the world, regarded as an economical raw material for the production of a variety of products, including paper and cloth.

You won't find many who will remember, but during World War Two, American farmers were subsidized by the U.S. government to grow the stuff for the manufacture of rope for ships. This industrial species of hemp is quite different from *Cannabis sativa* and is unsuitable as a drug; you can smoke all the Navy rope you want and the almost nonexistent level of THC will never get you high, in fact probably will make you sick enough to want to throw yourself off the side of the ship.*

Third, *ganja* was embraced for religious reasons. The anthropologist Weston La Barre dates cannabis use back to the Mesolithic period (Middle Stone Age) as part of a religious-shamanic belief system. Its use among the Islamic mystical order of Sufis (called by one rather irreverent historian "the hippies of the Arab world") is well documented. Hemp also had an important function in the mythology and present day ritual and ceremony of Shinto, or the "Way of the Gods," as the ancient indigenous religion of Japan is known. For the Rastafarians in Jamaica and the Sadhus in India, it is a religious sacrament, and it is so important to the Hindu religion that it was described in the *Atharva Veda* as a sacred grass, and the guardian angel of mankind is supposed to reside in its leaves. Buddhists, Zoroastrians, the ancient Israeli Essenes, and early Jews included the plant in their faith. There are even some Christians who believe the sacred "green herb of the field" in the Bible ("I will raise up for them a plant of renown, and they shall be no more consumed with hunger in the land, neither bear the shame of the heathen any more." Ezekiel 34:29) and the Biblical secret and sweet incenses and anointing oils to be cannabis. Tell that to George Bush and his friends in your dreams!

My interest is primarily in the fourth and final area, ma-

---

* The weird thing is that this kind of hemp is illegal most places, too.

rijuana's medicinal use. (Although the plant's function as a mood elevator and enhancer surely is related when it comes to sex.) For more than fifty years, religious and political conservatives, mainly in the U.S., have led a worldwide campaign to suppress the plant's use, despite an overwhelming body of scientific study finding cannabis far less harmful than caffeine, tobacco, and alcohol. Some of the bans have been removed in recent years, notably in the treatment of AIDS and glaucoma patients for whom it respectively serves as an appetite booster and pain reliever. It further has proved effective in reducing nausea for cancer patients undergoing radiation therapy. Still, it is in Asia where its use to treat a variety of ills goes—without interruption—back to 2000 BC. Recognizing this longstanding belief and codification of the plant's use, none of the UN Conventions related to drugs forbid medicinal use of cannabis (or, for that matter, opium).

Nowhere is this more evident than in modern India, where folk medicine practitioners representing the traditional Ayurveda, Siddha, and Unani (all Hindu) and Tibbi (Mohammedan) systems of medicine provide virtually all of the health care available in most of India's half million poor villages. It is especially in the Ayurvedic tradition where *bhang* (the dried mature leaves and flowering tops of both male and female plants) and *ganja* (the dried and resinous flowering tops of female plants only) are prescribed, for their sedative effect and stress reduction, as an appetite stimulant and digestive, as an anti-phlegmatic, and to treat a variety of diverse illnesses including fever, chronic diarrhea, rheumatism, conjunctivitis, swollen joints, gonorrhea, and malaria.

However much Western medicine may disagree with some of this treatment, there is a strong argument supporting the role of traditional practitioners, at least until university trained doctors are available in sufficient numbers and are willing to work in villages. It is for this reason that India's Narcotic Drugs and Psychotropic Substance Act (1985) not only permits *ganja*'s use for treatment of human ills (as well as to treat animals), but also mandates the government to establish a mechanism to supply cannabis to pharmaceutical companies and registered medical practitioners.

China's endorsement of the pot plant is less enthusiastic. The earliest known Chinese pharmacopoeia, the *Pen Ching*, dating from the first century BC and containing much older information, said, "To take too much makes people see demons and throw themselves about like maniacs. But if one takes it over a long period of time, one can communicate with the spirits and one's own body becomes light."

Despite numerous other Chinese references, cannabis has not played a comparable role in Chinese social life to that achieved in the Middle East and India. And it is in India where the believers and consumers reside in their greatest number today; it is here the plant is found growing wild throughout the Himalaya foothills and the adjoining plains, from Kashmir in the west to Assam in the east, flourishing even in the warm climate of the vast nation's tropical southern tip.

Given the millennia-long history of cannabis use in religious ceremony, it may be surprising that there is no mention of it in the *Ayurveda* prior to the eighth century AD. But there's no absence of cannabis in the long list of concoctions now, several of which are not only mixed and administered by the TSM practitioners—many of whom have up to twenty years of training—but also are sold openly in shops. One, called *Madana Modaka*, is sold in the form of "globlets" in vendor huts near schools and is purchased by schoolboys who want to get high. Yet, *Madana Modaka* is also a legitimate medicinal preparation in Ayurvedic practice, prescribed and marketed as a sexual stimulant as well as for flatulence and loss of appetite—its ingredients being cannabis leaves and seeds fried in ghee, along with numerous local herbs such as *thipal, kottan,* coriander, *asmodagam,* and *namal renu.*

"Cannabis is an essential ingredient in Ayurvedic treatment and we use it as a stimulant for patients recovering from paralysis and nerve-related illnesses, and as a sexual energizer for impotency," said Vidya Nidi Dr. K. Sayakkara, secretary of the All Ceylon Ayurvedic Practitioners' Congress. Ceylon (Sri Lanka) has sixteen thousand Ayurvedic practitioners and the laws and customs governing their use are almost identical to India's.

A study was made of the *Ayurveda,* along with other Indian texts, in 2001 by the United Nations Office on Drugs and Crime (UNODC), whose authors, Dr. I.C. Chopra, a pharmacologist, and Col. Sir R.N. Chopra of the World Health Organization, said, "In moderate doses, cannabis is believed to promote sexual desire and it is not an uncommon practice among the younger newly married folk to drink beverages and eat sweets containing *bhang.*" The authors then described some "Modes of Consumption," should anyone back in UN Headquarters in New York want recipes.

"The simplest *bhang* beverage consists of a drink made by pounding *bhang* leaves with a little black pepper and sugar, and diluting with water to the desired strength. Various kinds of special beverages are prepared by the middle and well-to-do classes by the addition of almonds, sugar, iced milk, curds, etc. A number of other ingredients are often added to improve the taste and with the idea of enhancing the euphoric effect of the beverage. Among these ingredients, aniseed, *ajawan,* cucumber, melon and poppy seeds, rose petals, saffron, cloves, cardamom and musk are the most common. Pistachio nuts, asafetida, liquorice, senna leaves and extracts derived from various other herbs are not infrequently added. Fruit juices such as those derived from pomegranate, date palm and bael fruit and also coconut milk form ingredients for such drinks. Besides improving the taste, these spices and flavorings are popularly believed to counteract the harmful effects of the regular use of cannabis drugs."

It didn't stop there. Those wild and crazy Chopras went on to tell how to make *majun,* "a special type of confection on the preparation of which *bhang* or, very occasionally, *ganja,* is either heated in a little *ghee* (clarified butter) or boiled in water. The active resin, which is lighter, floats to the surface in the form of a green, jelly-like substance. This greenish scum is separated, then mixed with sugar and heated over a fire to form a paste that on settling is cut into small pieces. This is eaten on the same day or within a few days of its preparation."

Recipes for *halva* (the Middle Eastern, Central Asian and Indian sweet) and curry followed.

Elsewhere in the report the authors summarized what it called "Sexual Factors," saying that cannabis was "perhaps the cheapest and most easily procurable of all narcotic drugs that have been taken by mankind with the idea of obtaining pleasurable sensation and stimulation of their sexual appetite."

At last, I thought, the money given by the world's governments to the UN was being wisely spent.

One Consumer's Endorsement

"The only aphrodisiac I can vouch for is pot," wrote a friend when I sent email messages to everyone in my address book asking help when I started writing this book.

"It always works for me," she said. "I just wish they would isolate that part of it, so you could use it when you want to fuck, but don't want to get high."

Chapter ten
The Other Story of O

I experimented with drugs in the 1960s, but never played with heroin or any other opium derivatives. It wasn't until I moved to Thailand, a country that provided one corner of the infamous "Golden Triangle" of nations (the others being Laos and Burma), that I thought about going to the source.

And not to get high, but hard.

Because opium, the resinous goop that is harvested from the delicate poppy plant, was known in much of the Middle and Far East a couple of hundred years ago—especially in China and India—as an effective aphrodisiac. Before I describe my trek into the hill tribe villages of the Golden Triangle region, a few words about how this came about.

The geographical origin of the opium poppy (*Papaver somniferum*, its Latin name giving it a sleepy connation) is not certain, but it is thought to be in Europe; poppy remains have been found in archeological excavations in Switzerland, southern Germany, and southern England going back four thousand years. However, most of the earliest historical references come from the Middle East, where as early as 2,500 BC Assyrian medical texts referred to it as "The Plant of Joy." The poppy and opium also were both sacred to many of the Greek gods and much later it was added, along with a member of the nightshade family, to the wine of Cleopatra.

Traders from the Arab states are credited with taking the plant to India where it was embraced by the systems of Unani and Ayurvedic medicine. The first reference in the latter comes from the thirteenth century, when it was described as a *vajikarana* (aphrodisiac). The ingredients in one blend included equal parts of eight different plants and herbs (including ginger, cubeb pepper, nutmeg, clove, and sandalwood) and four parts *ahiphena* (opium). It was said that men who took the powdered mixture during the day would be loved by women at night.

Opium also gained favor as an analgesic and soporific, but its primary use was to halt premature ejaculation, prolong erection, and increase erotic pleasure. Frequently it was taken with *ganja, charas* or hashish and, as with Cleopatra, nightshade. The lovely flower and the dried sap that oozed from the incised seedpod also was consecrated to Shiva, the shaman god of Ecstasy and inner vision, the third member of the Hindu trinity, along with Brahma and Vishnu.

Yet it was in China where opium truly blossomed, becoming, as Christian Räatsch wrote in *Plants of Love*, "a veritable symbol of sex. Pressed into the shape of small fish, it was sold under the name *ying-tsu-su*. The Chinese expression 'fish and water come together' refers to sexual intercourse. In ancient China, the word 'fish' had the symbolic meaning of 'penis'." Further, in the ancient erotic novel *Dschau-yang dschii-schii* (*The Golden Lord Mounts the White Tiger*) it was said opium would give life to a tired lance, assuring at least three thousand thrusts.

It was also in China in more modern times—as well as across much of what was then called Indochine (Laos, Cambodia, and Vietnam), the East Indies (Indonesia), and as far north as Taiwan—that smoking opium far overwhelmed the taking of the resin internally. Here, during the Ming (1358–1644) and early Qing (1644–1911) dynasties the opium poppy became one of the most important plants in China's history.

Zheng Yangwen of the National University of Singapore, author of *The Social Life of Opium in China* (2005), approached the consumption of opium in terms of social and class differences. He said opium was an aristocratic luxury during the Ming dynasty, so "its vanguard consumers, the literati and officials, enjoyed opium long before the 'ordinary' people heard about it. It was they who made opium smoking cultured and a status symbol; they who marked themselves apart from those below them, legitimating their social differences.

"An opium pipe carved with an epic poem and served by a highly literate courtesan was limited to and had meaning for those who could appreciate the poetry and exchange coded language."

Opium's use as a medicinal remedy thus was supplanted by its consumption as something to enhance sex for emperors and their consorts. Vassal states presented opium to the Ming court as a tribute. When the great eunuch-admiral Zheng He set forth on his first voyage in 1405, going as far as Africa to the west (and, some believe, the North American continent to the east), opium was considered a fitting gift from poppy-growing states to send back to China in much the same way gifts are exchanged today between heads of state.

The plant's elitist status continued into the early Qing dynasty, when it continued to be a key part of the upper class's sex recreation, but long before the last emperor was shuttled aside by China's first republican leaders in 1911, its use and standing executed a one-hundred-eighty-degree turn. In the early nineteenth century, opium made its way from the top down to the middle and lower classes, changing the phrase "social status" to "social problem" and then political crisis.

England was in great debt to China because it imported more tea, silk, and porcelain than it could offset by its meager sale of wool and spices, and China insisted on up-front payment in silver. So the British East-India Company planted huge poppy plantations in Bengal and started sending opium to China, selling it illegally. In 1838, China struck back, destroying 2.64 million pounds (1.2 million kilograms) of opium in Canton (now Guangzhou). This triggered the first "Opium War" and after two years, China accepted Britain's demands—compensation for the destroyed opium, open trade, and the handover of Hong Kong. (The East India Company's principal agent at the time was Jardin Matheson; now you know how the present day multinational got its start.) When the emperor refused to honor this treaty, the British moved in again, training its guns on Nanjing. China finally surrendered.

Chinese use of opium continued and the "opium den" became as unfortunate a cliché connected to China, in the West anyway, as Chinese restaurants and laundries. Such emporiums of dream and joy also continued into the twentieth century in northern Burma and Thailand, Indochina, and Taiwan.

The simple pipes were made from a long piece of bamboo with a metal bowl, into which was placed a small "pill" of opium. The smoker usually lay on his side on a mat or opium "bed," preparation of the pipe traditionally carried out in the better parlors by women whose role was somewhat similar to that of the geisha in Japan, and in some of the cheaper places by small boys who were, on demand, also catamites.

The Encyclopedia of Sex Practice (publication date unknown) states, "Opium smoking induces strange sexual fantasies which are associated with the sense of voluptuous pleasure, and for a time it also produces erection, though after continual use this effect ceases and, indeed, continued opium smoking eventually leads to total impotence. In women, too, opium smoking intensifies the sexual instinct to a considerable extent…" This is confirmed in a French text, *Manuel des Maladies des Voies Urinaires* (publication date unknown), urging small doses. When ten to twelve pipes are taken, it was said that "any suggestion of erotic excitement in the individual, whether by direct contact or merely by mental image, immediately produces an erection.* Despite this, however, the penile nerves, especially those of the glans, become anesthetized, with the result that orgasm and emission is considerably retarded. A similar effect is produced in the female (vulva, vagina, and rectal nerves being anesthetized). The rectal and vaginal constrictor muscles become relaxed. Under this condition, pederasty has been practiced more easily, and without pain, despite an obvious anatomical disproportion."

In all the literature there is talk of an Ultimate Aphrodisiac and one often mentioned is the "Oriental Joy

---

* Perhaps explaining Graham Greene's comment in *Ways of Escape* (1980) that of the four winters he spent in Indochine, it was opium that "left the happiest memory."

Pill." However corny its name, apparently it did (and may still) exist. Christian Räatsch is vague about its country of origin, waffling between India and China, although China gets the nod in other sources, including one published in Europe in the early nineteenth century.

"To dispel a bad mood and hypochondriac disturbances, the Orientals, who are known to take delight in smoking and eating opium, take their refuge in a mixture called nepenthe, which consists of the powder of the dried topmost leaves and flowers of hemp, together with opium, areca nut, spices, and sugar, which they swallow in pill form." Räatsch quoted another source as saying, "The seeds [of the thorn apple] also comprise an ingredient of the Oriental joy pill, which contains poppy juice, hemp, and several spices as well; for the Oriental, who is forbidden wine, this is a surrogate for the same and is said to evoke an indescribable sense of well-being…"

I hadn't even heard of Räatsch and the Oriental Joy Pill when, in the middle 1990s, I was researching a book about the Hmong, one of the more colorful ethnic minorities in Asia, known mainly in modern times for their participation in the secret war in Laos against the Pathet Lao and Viet Cong during America's war with Vietnam. But I had heard, from friends, about what they called the "friendly" effects of opium.

A "hill tribe" that originated in southern China and over centuries moved into Laos, northern Thailand and Vietnam in the nineteenth century, the Hmong were known for their skill in growing the opium poppy—using the opium themselves mainly as an all-purpose medication and selling off the surplus, most of which was processed by others into heroin. At the time of my arrival in Hmong territory, it was illegal to cultivate, market or consume opium and its byproducts virtually everywhere in the world, but of course that didn't change the agricultural reality, it only drove the price up, and the main countries of origin in the 1990s were Afghanistan, Burma, and Laos. It also was being grown in smaller commercial quantity in China, India, Vietnam, and North Korea. A few years later Burma took the Number One position when the Taleban cracked down in Afghanistan. After the U.S. "liberated" that country, Afghanistan went back to the top of the list of opium producing countries.

Anyway, in 1995, when I was researching my book about the Hmong, a crop substitution program was under way to knock out the last of its cultivation in Thailand, sponsored by His Majesty Adulyadej Bhumibol and supported by the U.S. through its Drug Enforcement Agency (DEA). Visiting the many remote Hmong villages in my study of the culture, it was clear that the campaign to replace the poppy with potatoes and apricots at that time still had a way to go.

As I entered the small highland hamlet a couple of hours from Chiang Mai, traveling by hired motorbike and then on foot, I saw about thirty rustic homes arranged in what I knew was a precise pattern, to permit the spirits easy passage through the village, thus rendering them unthreatening. The structures were no more than huts, with bamboo and roughly hewn wood walls, aged in appearance with lots of wide cracks, hard dirt floors, and a coarse roof thatched with dried leaves. Pigs and chickens and naked children roamed freely in the dust. An old woman was bent over a tub coloring cloth made from hemp grown in a nearby garden. Her hands and wrists were a dark blue from the indigo dye, made from a plant grown in the same garden. Another old woman sat at a loom, weaving. It was mid-day and most of the younger adults were in the fields, lancing the opium buds, collecting the sap, and keeping an eye out for the cops and DEA.

I had been to this village before, but I still wasn't permitted a visit to the fields, created some distance away in the traditional slash-and-burn manner. There, I knew, just a few weeks earlier, the white, crimson, and mauve blossoms had fallen away and now the villagers were moving from plant to plant with tapping tools consisting of a set of three or four parallel metal blades mounted on a handle. Each bud was sliced two or three times, to allow the sticky sap to flow. Each day, this "latex" was collected on a knife that was wetted (with water or by the harvester's tongue) so the sap wouldn't stick to the blade, and placed in a container worn around his or her waist.

The opium was dried in the sun and "cooked" in boiling water, then left to simmer until all that remained was a thick, brown paste. This was pressed into molds or trays and dried again in the sun until it had the consistency of dense modeling clay. Now it was ready to smoke.

With the village headman's nod of approval, I was offered a pipe. This wasn't a big deal in the 1990s because many villages were providing opium to tourists as part of a hill tribe visit, organized by trekking companies in Chiang Mai. But this village wasn't one of them and I felt honored to have been given approval to rest on a bamboo platform inside one of the huts and smoke with one of the older men.

The pipe was prepared and the pinhead-sized ball of opium was ignited with a taper lit from the single candle that provided the only illumination. I inhaled deeply and slowly released the smoke through my nostrils. I coughed. The old man near me smiled and nodded in what appeared to be encouragement.

A second bowl was prepared. That prompted a full-on coughing fit. I rested for a short while, enjoying the peace that washed over me, waiting for the visions, the sexual fantasies that my friends had told me about, the erection promised by some of the texts.

A third bowl was prepared. Again I inhaled deeply. And I vomited.

Opium contains sugars, proteins, ammonia, latex, gums, plant wax, fats, sulphuric and lactic acids, water, meconic acid, and a wide range of alkaloids. The key parts of the mix are the fifty or more alkaloids, the most important being morphine, from which codeine and heroin are made. That, reportedly, is what incites sexual excitement.

Opiates may be swallowed, smoked, injected, sniffed, inhaled, or absorbed through mucous membranes. Today, opium is rarely smoked anywhere in Asia, because, like cannabis, it is illegal to sell or possess and, in some countries, the punishment is exceedingly harsh. It's also a lot of trouble, the ritual too complex to appeal to many.

(Historic items connected to opium draw big prices, however. There is a lucrative market for antique opium beds, some of the more elaborately carved and decorated ones selling for thousands of dollars in Hong Kong and Taipei. The weights used for measuring opium, metallic roosters and the like, are a popular item for Asian collectors. And for the tourist, a replica of an opium pipe—its stem solid, thus making it unusable and easier to take through customs—is a wonderful souvenir to take home from China, Cambodia, or Vietnam.)

If opium were legal, there would be many commercial benefits. Poppy seeds may be used as a condiment with baked goods and pastries for their nutty odor and flavor (reminiscent of almonds). Poppy seed oil has been widely used in cooking, in the manufacture of perfumes and, because of its drying properties, as a base for expensive artists' oil paints. It has been used as an antispasmodic, diaphoretic, expectorant, hypnotic, and sedative, as well as to kill pain.

As for getting the old man up again, or at least delivering enchanting, sexual fantasies, perhaps I'll never know.

Chapter eleven
The Placebo Effect

The phrase could've been the title of a novel by Robert Ludlum. This is appropriate, because "the placebo effect" is as much a mystery as were *The Bourne Identity*, *The Osterman Weekend*, and *The Sigma Protocol*.

One of my dictionaries defines the placebo—Latin for "I shall please"—as "the phenomenon that a patient's symptoms can be alleviated by an otherwise ineffective treatment, apparently because the individual *expects* or *believes* that it will work." And in a book called *Follies and Fallacies in Medicine* (1990), Petr Skrabanek and James McCormick say, "The physician's belief in the treatment and the patient's faith in the physician exert a reinforcing effect; the result is a powerful remedy that is almost guaranteed to produce an improvement and sometimes a cure."

Most of us think of placebos as substances such as sugar or starch given to some of the subjects in so-called double-blind studies of new drugs, in which neither the subjects nor the researchers know who is getting what. The theory is that if as many subjects improve by taking the placebo as do by taking the chemical concoction, then the drug being tested is regarded as a failure and probably on its way to the dustbin.

Other times, the use of placebos is recommended. There is even "placebo surgery" now, where patients with real symptoms are anesthetized and cut and stitched up again, with nothing done inside. How can that be? It's done because placebos often work.

According to an article in the *New York Times Magazine* in 1999, the "bigger and more dramatic the patient perceives the intervention to be, the bigger the placebo effect." The writer went on to say that between thirty-five and seventy-five per cent of patients benefited from taking a dummy pill in studies of new drugs. So that what we had here, the writer said, was "benign deception" that turned into "lies that heal."

Some credit the nature-taking-its-course theory, believing that at least part of the placebo's apparent good effect is due to the fact that we often heal spontaneously if we do nothing at all, that illness waxes and wanes and sometimes goes into remission. Others say the emotional alliance between doctor and patient that emerges from an atmosphere of hope actually does relieve stress, and that this, in turn, leads to a change in attitude and that this may, in fact, alter one's body chemistry.

Cynics call it self-deception or wishful thinking. Skeptics say it's the power of positive thinking. True believers insist it's a miracle.

And so it may be with numerous so-called aphrodisiacs. Starting with most if not all of the liquids and capsules and pills marketed on the Internet by the countless thousands of greedy descendants of the "snake oil salesmen" who traveled the American west in wagons in the nineteenth century, selling miracle cures that mostly contained a lot of alcohol. Go online and type in the word "aphrodisiacs," as I did, and in about a tenth of a second of wait time, Google delivered 2,550,000 pages for me to look at.

Walk into an apothecary in India or China or any big-city Chinatown or any *apotek* in Indonesia and how many herbs and packaged pills will you find guaranteed to make you strong? The choice is staggering, in both the traditional shops where there are walls of drawers full of dried bone and plants that are measured and mixed on the spot, and in the snazzy modern ones where everything is prepackaged and sold on open shelves.

Ever since hearing about Xingshijiu, the herbal remedy from Shanghai with Viagra's magic ingredient *sildenafil citrate* secretly and illegally added, I wanted to try it. I asked a friend who had a joint venture business in Shanghai to see if he could find some next time he went there. My friend has an avid curiosity and an active sense of humor, so he spent the better part of a day searching and while he didn't find the stuff, he bought a sack full of other goodies that he was told would do the trick, along with a story to tell.

David admits his Mandarin isn't good, so he took two of the young Chinese who work for him in Shanghai along on his visit to a couple of dozen shops. One was a translator, the other a graphics designer, and both were young Chinese women. Now, you have to picture David, who is a fifty-something American and built along the lines of a sumo wrestler, asking for aphrodisiacs while standing there with two local women who are half his age and a third his weight. Of course, he said he was conducting his search for a friend who was writing a book. How many do you think believed him?

Anyway, he returned to Bangkok with more than twenty boxes of he and I knew not what, English appearing on the beautifully designed packages as rarely as it was spoken in the shops where he bought the stuff. Most, I assumed, were the slow-acting sex boosters of the sort suggested by most Traditional Chinese Medicine practitioners, to be taken regularly for several months before expecting any clear result. I didn't have that kind of time to devote to any field testing I would otherwise be willing to try—and couldn't take more than one at a time in any case, for fear of their conflicting—so I focused on the ones where there was some promise offered by my friend's oral report or the ingredients identified on the packaging (in rare English) that seemed to offer more immediate effect.

David bought two boxes of something called Weikang, he said, because the pharmacist said it was as good as Cialis. I looked at the contents and, sure enough, the pills inside were diamond-shaped. Inside, in Chinese, Japanese, Korean, and English was a list of ingredients: spirulina (the algae-based food supplement that I guess gave the pills their green color), arillus longan, almonds, licorice, fructus mori, fructose lycil, poria, and mulberry leaf. They seemed an innocent lot of plants, but, who knew? I swallowed one.

You can guess what happened. Nothing.

I took another. More of the same.

I was next drawn to an atomizer containing what was described as "Male Regeneration Distillate Dew" because it listed *damiana* and *yohimbé* as two of its ingredients. (This was another one of the few with English labeling.) I knew that the bark of the *yohimbé* tree in west Africa was the world's most effective male sexual stimulant; everyone on the planet is in agreement about this—and *damiana*, a tropical plant that grows from Mexico to the Seychelles to parts of Asia, usually came along in second place—the leaves dried and finely pulverized and commonly taken in capsule form.

It was the mention of *yohimbé* that raised my hopes, though not my expectations. The Food and Drug Administration in my home country approved it to dilate (widen) the pupils of eyes, but the FDA also said in 1995 that it found little or no *yohimbine* in eleven of eighteen brands of *yohimbé* supplements sold on the open marketplace. Still, I knew that since *yohimbé* caused blood vessels to dilate and blood flow to increase, many physicians prescribed it for ED.

The "dew" was contained in a gracefully curving atomizer labeled "Borost," which I took to be the manufacturer's name, as on both the atomizer and outer box were the following words (appearing here exactly as they appeared): "The Borost professor and experts made more Than thousand experiments, finally successfully extracted. Yohimbé which can regenerate the sponge cell of the male genitals from Damiana leaves. E.S the plant regeneration element. After six years researching, Borost and other 13 male procreation experts of the U.S. finally discovered a king of green plant called Damiana by indigenes in North-America. As early as before 16 centuries indigenes discovered that after bull eat this kind of plant, its procreation ability becomes especially strong."

Assuming (somewhat capriciously) that what I held in my hand actually contained *damiana* and *yohimbé* and because my reference books all said they were consumed orally, I further assumed that the "mist" was to be sprayed onto my tongue or into my open mouth. So that's what I did. One, two, three small hits. There was a taste and smell of cheap cologne—something I would not normally put on the outside of my face, let alone inside it—that lingered for, maybe, twenty minutes. And then I waited. And waited. And waited.

I tried it again the next day, this time taking six hits. (I live in Bangkok where a lot of people speak and read Chinese, I told myself, so why didn't I get someone to translate the instructions inside the box? Maybe it suggested ten hits. Or, maybe, only one.) Again, I waited.

Imagine it. Here I am, alone in my apartment in Bangkok (my wife in our country home an eight-hour train ride away), a borrowed X-rated DVD providing some proxy lasciviousness, flesh on standby, drinking beer to get rid of the cloying, perfumey taste, and really, truly hoping the damned stuff will work.

I concluded that the Chinese were either lousy chemists or good liars. And was reminded of a story I pulled off the Net from a Chinese website, *China.org.cn*, by Li Liangdu in 2003 warning shoppers to beware.

"Promotional materials are sensational and make exaggerated claims for the products. Fake addresses are given for the 'suppliers.' Imported goods including medicines are sold without the benefit of Chinese translations or the instructions for their safe use. Dates of manufacture are a mystery and of course some sort of guarantee would be quite out of the question. Even worse, some stores sell outdated or fake medicines with the accompanying risk of serious health problems.

"Ironically, this is one group of customers unlikely to pursue justice in the courts if they become victims of these poor quality products. Nor do they take their complaints to the consumers' associations. Well, they wouldn't, would they?

"So far there is no single official body with a specific remit to set standards for, or to monitor the manufacture, sale and quality of products in this relatively recently emerging market. Those responsibilities that do exist are made less effective by being spread across the boundaries between and among several different government departments. Consequently there are loopholes to be exploited by both manufacturers and retailers."

But that mouth spray could have worked, yes?

Perhaps if I'd had more faith.

Chapter twelve
Cruel & Unusual Aphrodisia

On a visit to Vientiane, the capital of Laos, in late 2005, I saw someone handing out flyers to passersby and slipping them under the windscreen wipers on parked cars. A man ahead of me glanced at the one he was given, crumpled it up in obvious displeasure and discarded it. When I reached the man with the flyers, he did not offer one. I held out my hand.

"For Lao," he said. He showed me the flyer. Whatever he was selling was described in the local language. I went back and picked up the flyer that lay discarded on the road and later that day, meeting a Lao friend for drinks, I showed it to him.

"It's for a bear farm," he said. "I didn't know there was one in Laos. Usually you find them in China."

I had heard, and read, about bear farms. The use of bear parts in Chinese medicine went back thousands of years and since the 1980s the precious bile believed to be effective in treating a variety of illnesses, as well as increasing sexual energy, had been "milked" from live bears on "farms." These were places where the animals were kept in long rows of cages; a metal or rubber catheter was surgically inserted into the bile duct or gall bladder, a technique developed in South Korea that quickly spread to China and Vietnam.

The World Society for the Protection of Animals (WSPA) was quoted in an exhaustive book on the subject, *The Bear Bile Business* (2002), as saying originally there were many small farms, but in recent years there had been a consolidation that resulted in fewer farms holding more bears. In 1998, the society stated matter-of-factly, that that left 247 farms with 7,002 bears. Another source said there were another 4,000 on farms in Vietnam. I checked with a friend who works at the London Zoo and he referred me to some websites and it appears that there are perhaps ten times as many bears in cages on farms than in all of the zoos in the world!

"The commercialization of the bear trade during the last twenty years has seen huge quantities of bear bile produced, far in excess of what can be consumed in China," the WSPA went on. "Therefore, external markets are keenly sought despite the fact that it is illegal to export the product. It has been claimed that bear farming would help bear conservation. However, despite the presence of farmed bear bile, the gall from a wild bear is seen as more potent and is worth considerably more. Therefore, there is significant poaching of wild bears, not only in Asia, but globally."

What further galled the WSPA (sorry for the pun) was the fact that in 1955, Japanese scientists succeeded in synthesizing Ursodeoxycholic acid (UDCA), the active ingredient in bear bile that was believed to have beneficial medicinal effect. Today, large quantities of UDCA are made synthetically from cow bile and are widely used in Western medicine to dissolve gallstones and treat cirrhosis of the liver. It's estimated that about 45,000 pounds (100,000 kg) of the synthetic is being consumed each year in China, Japan, and South Korea, and that the world figure may be double this. No one knows how much of "the real thing" is consumed, although one thing is certain: there are consumers who believe it is more powerful and they are willing to pay for it. It is for this reason, surely, that so many dead bears are found in the wild—and not just in Asia, but also in North America—with only their gall bladders (and perhaps their paws) removed.

In 1999 and 2000, the WSPA visited eleven Chinese bear farms—called "bruin concentration camps" by another NGO—and found "barren housing, poor hygiene and nutrition, improper surgery and veterinary care, early weaning and maternal separation [of younger bears from their mothers, who were returned soon after breeding to the milking cage]." Until recently, the bile continuously drained into a plastic sac and in others, the tube was opened and the bladder was drained once or twice daily. This method of bile extraction continues on most smaller farms, but has been replaced on others where the animal is knocked out with a veterinary tranquilizer called Ketamine, the gall bladder is located by ultrasound, and the green bile is sucked out with a large hypodermic needle, once every three or four months. The two hundred and fifty cubic centimeters produced in one milking in 2004 sold for about $1,000.

However cruel and bizarre bear farming may sound to those elsewhere, in China it was no big thing. In fact, the Chinese government actually licensed the businesses and designated some of them "model government farms." The Chinese had a history of farming wildlife. In the 1950s, musk deer farms sprang up to meet growing demand for musk oil. Subsequently, breeding programs were started for tigers, civets, pangolins, flying squirrels, snakes, turtles, frogs, toads, scorpions, and various types of fish and insects. And in Vietnam, where bear farming is officially banned, it is nonetheless regarded as a part of an unstated government policy to create employment opportunities for rural communities.

Products made from farmed bear bile include powders, capsules, ointments, tablets, tinctures, suppositories, eye drops, throat lozenges, cough syrup, hemorrhoid cream, wines, teas, shampoos, and tonics. The products were expensive, but WSPA found pharmacies carrying them in Indonesia, Japan, Malaysia, Singapore, Taiwan, Australia, Canada, and the U.S.

My friend in Vientiane translated the flyer and said the farm offered free pickup and return and for those who wanted to drink the bile "directly from live bear," that was possible, too. My friend continued to read from the flyer: "Paper say, 'We suck bear bile every Saturday and Sunday. Guarantee quality one hundred per cent with negotiate price, one cubic centimeter only 150,000 kip ($15).'"

I said I wanted to go.

He laughed. "Never happen," he said. "*You farang*. Think you NGO."

Enormous cruelty is inflicted on creatures great and small in the interest of improving sex. Many of us saw Harrison Ford offered fresh monkey brains in the 1984 movie *Indiana Jones and the Temple of Doom*, when a live monkey was strapped beneath a table with a hole in the center, then had its skull cap deftly removed, whereupon Mr. Jones was handed a spoon. I don't recall where that scene was supposed to have taken place, or even if the location was identified, but I've been assured by a photographer friend in Hong Kong that for several hundred U.S. dollars, such a live, warm meal could be prepared on order in southern China today. This is a story I did not pursue.

As it happens, much nastiness occurs frequently in the pursuit of increasing sexual strength. In Hanoi, I was told about the breaking of dogs' legs before killing them for a stir-fry and in Thailand I heard about lowering live bears in cages so their feet go into a pot of boiling water or onto a bed or glowing coals before they are chopped off and cooked up in a soup. (That costs anywhere from $60 in Thailand to $1,000 overseas.)

Why?

In a single word: adrenaline. When adrenaline is released into the bloodstream at times of fear and anxiety, the heart beats faster, the central nervous system is stimulated, male hormones called androgens are released, and, for some reason that culinary science has not yet explored (nor is likely to), there are many who believe that the meat's taste and therapeutic effect is enhanced.

I once had a conversation with someone who didn't condone breaking legs and lowering bears into hot water, mind you, but he asked how different was it from letting live fish flop around in a plastic tub with only an inch of water in it, as is common in Asia's open markets? Or throwing live chickens and ducks into metal drums of boiling water to loosen their feathers before plucking, another common marketplace sight? And how different was that, he asked, from the Western custom of casually dumping live crabs and lobsters into boiling water?

By then, I'd heard enough, but the guy wasn't finished. Had I ever been to a slaughterhouse? he asked. I told him that I had, many times. Why did I think it was called that? Did I think that when someone banged those creatures over the head with a metal pipe and slit their throats, they were being "put to sleep," as Westerners often euphemized death?

"Alright, alright," I said, "enough."

But it wasn't enough.

There was still the story of the poacher to be told. What's called "poaching" now used to be called "hunting" and it was part of the hunter-gatherer's everyday means of survival, going back to prehistoric times when surely most of the killing of animals was to feed the family or community and if there was anything left over, it was sold or bartered for other goods. Offer a villager $40 today for a pangolin, the indigenous anteater whose blood is valued in Asia as an aphrodisiac, when that sum equals perhaps a month's earnings at hard labor, and it's difficult to mistake why the guy sets traps for pangolin.

Such men are now called poachers because they're killing endangered species—often in national parks—and many of them are part of a huge international network of traffickers who cater to a black market estimated by Interpol to be worth at least $6 billion a year.

One of the most valuable items is the rhinoceros horn, which has been used in traditional Asian medicine for an estimated two thousand years, most notoriously as an aphrodisiac. The reason cited most often had to do with the "law of similarity"; the horn sort of looked like a penis, therefore (the belief went) its consumption, ground into a powder, would make a man "strong."

Another reason for the animal's popularity was the rhino's sexual stamina. My friend at the London Zoo told me that for the black rhino, copulation lasts for twenty minutes at a time and continues for two to three days. "The female is unable to support the weight of the (usually bigger) male for too long," he said, "and will moan when she's had enough. And when he ejaculates, there are buckets of it."

Only five rhino species survive today, following a history that goes back fifty million years. There are about three thousand black and white rhinos in Africa, a sorry number compared to the 65,000 to 100,000 that roamed the continent under fifty years ago. The picture is no brighter in Asia, where one of the major differences is that Asian rhinos share their range with a high density of people. The development of agriculture required to feed the exploding population has resulted in the loss of habitat. So where once the Indian rhino could be found from Pakistan across the northern part of the subcontinent to Bangladesh, and northward into Nepal and Bhutan, now they are confined to the swamps and riverine forests of the Terai and Brahmaputra Rivers. This species is by far the largest, weighing up to 5,900 pounds (2,700 kg), about the same as a new pickup truck.

The Sumatran rhinos range over Burma, Thailand, the Malaysian peninsula and on the islands of Sumatra and Java, but their numbers are small, down to perhaps ten in Thailand, with the largest population, two hundred, on the island of Sumatra. This is the smallest species, weighing up to 2,100 pounds (950 kg).

The Javan rhino is almost as big as the Indian, weighing as much as 5,000 pounds (2,300 kg), but its plight is the greatest, with only fifty or sixty believed left in the wild. So rare is this species, no zoo anywhere in the world even has one.

All have horns; the Sumatran species, two, and the densely matted hair (not bone) that comprises the broad-based, sharply pointed protrusion has been a valuable ingredient in

Traditional Chinese Medicine to treat fever, delirium, high blood pressure and other ailments. Today the use of rhino horn in TCM is banned throughout most of Asia, but before laws were introduced, hundreds of the animals were killed every year, and best estimates are that laws forbidding poaching haven't diminished the trade, only driven prices up—this, despite the fact that science says all the claims are false. After laboratory tests, Hoffman-La Roche, one of the world's largest pharmaceutical companies, declared that it had no effect on the human body whatsoever. Chinese scientists in Hong Kong found that rhino horn did have a cooling effect on fever—the other popular reason for its consumption—but only when used in massive doses.

Most of the poached animals were shot, the bodies left behind after the horns were removed with axes or saws. Others fell into pit traps and some were electrocuted after hunters tapped into high-tension power lines and strung the wire across trails as far as a kilometer away.

As rhino populations fell in both Africa and Asia, the horn's value grew to be worth more than five times its weight in gold. Ben Davies told a story in *Black Market: Inside the Endangered Species Trade in Asia* (2005) about a plot to drive the price even higher. In 1993, he said, a team of undercover investigators went after what he called "the world's most powerful rhino horn cartel."

Steve Galster of WildAid in Bangkok tracked a shipment of horns from Durban and Cape Town in South Africa to Taiwan, then the center for rhino horn smuggling. (Lacking UN recognition, Taiwan is not a signatory to international conservation treaties and parts from many endangered species have been sold there openly.) There, Galster found a stockpile estimated to total nine tons—the booty from 3,700

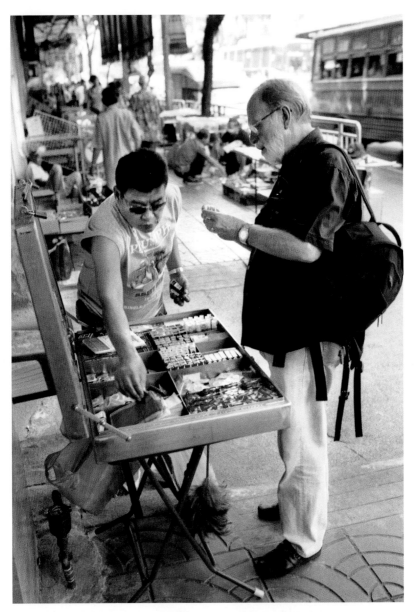

The author ponders a purchase from a sidewalk vendor of potions and lotions and sex aids in Bangkok's Chinatown. Identical stands are commonplace in many parts of Asia, the display cases designed so that if a cop approaches, the salesman can merely close the case and walk away. (Photo by Martin Reeves)

Aphrodisiacs take many forms, including a bottle of camphor-enhanced crocodile oil from Thailand, one of the more popular Viagra "clones" from India, a copy of an ornate silver hash pipe from Cambodia, some dried opium poppy buds from Laos, and a seahorse purchased in China. (Photos by Martin Reeves)

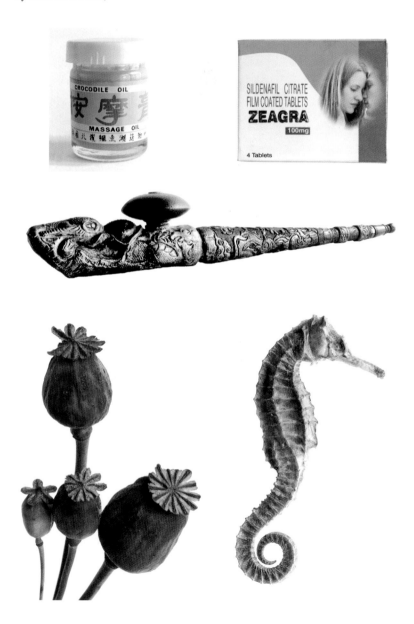

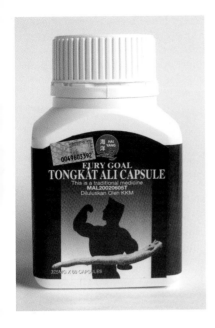

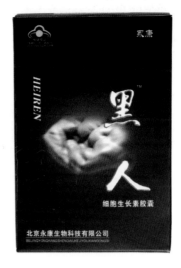

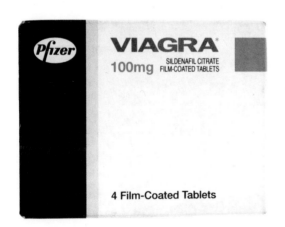

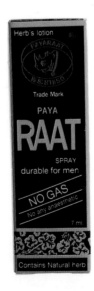

From Malaysia, a bottle of capsules containing Tongkat Ali root, a Chinese package with what appears to be a penis depicted, a four-pill box of Viagra (the aphrodisiac world's "real thing"), and an atomizer from Thailand with a rhino on the label, but none on the ingredient list, a spray for "durability." (Photos by Martin Reeves)

With the exception of the package containing blue Viagra "clones" (below left) and the box emblazoned by a drawing of an American Indian (center), both from China, all the packaged powders and pills shown were purchased in shops and on the street in Indonesia. Ancient gods, the horse, lion, and modern day muscle men are popular motifs, implying that consumption of the pills and capsules will make you "strong".
(Photos by Martin Reeves)

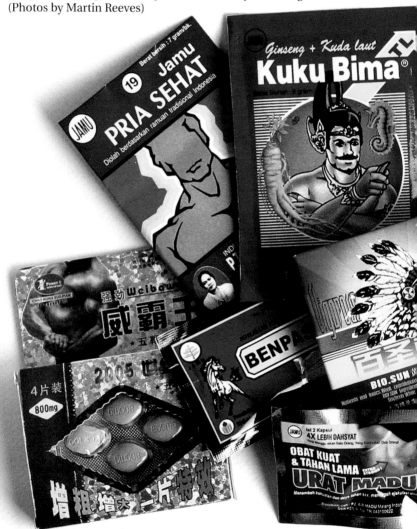

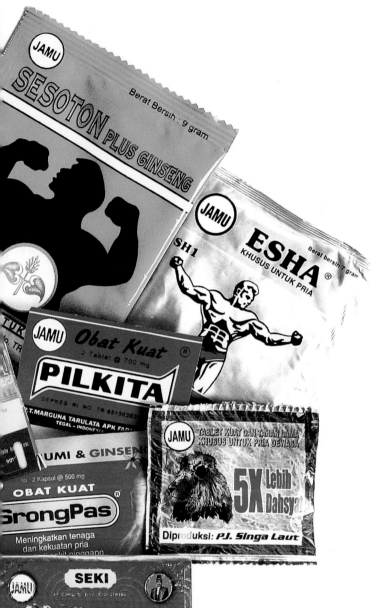
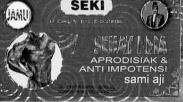

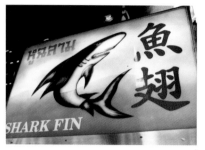

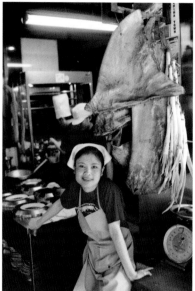

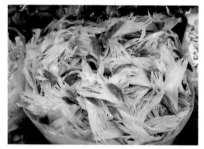

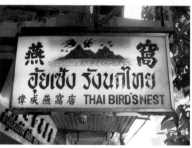

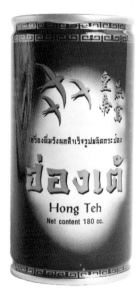

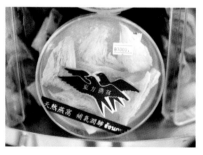

Signs advertising shark fin and bird's nest soup are common throughout China, in Thailand and Malaysia where the nests are harvested, and in Chinatowns everywhere. Often the largest fins are displayed, though most of the fins and nests end up shredded and dried or used in a canned drink. (Photos by Martin Reeves)

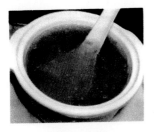

处女燕
Virgin Bird's Soup

润肺养颜、健脾开胃
Nourishes lungs & complexion,
stimulate appetite.

RM 280

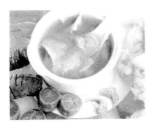

菩萨跳舞
Dancing Buddha Soup
(野泡参、花胶、鱼鳔、干贝、海参)
(American wild ginseng, fish maw, dried scallop,
sea cucumber)

提神补气、防骨疏松、软化血管
Strengthen "qi" ,improve bone density,
softening blood vessels.

RM 53

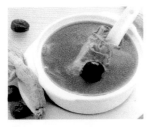

人参炖鸡 👍
Ginseng & Chicken Soup

提神、清热、行血
Stimulates physical vigour & blood circulation,
eliminates heat.

RM 25

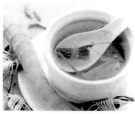

羚羊麦冬灯芯花
Antelope's Horn &
"Mak Dong" Soup
(孕妇忌食)
(Not recommended for pregnancy)

平肝熄火、清湿热、排毒
Eliminates heat,clears damp-heat & detox.

RM 22

Four aphrodisiac soups offered in Kuala Lumpur's Chinatown. (Photos by
Martin Reeves)

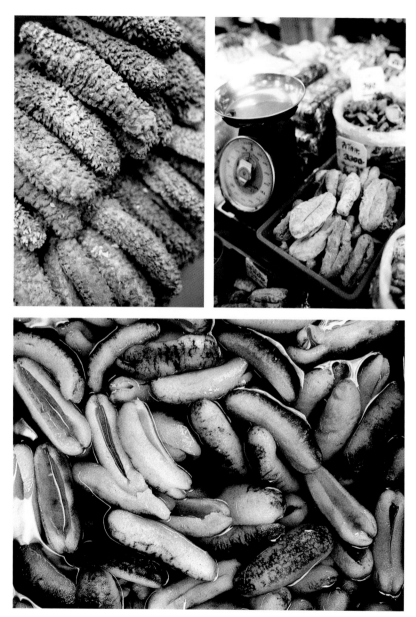

Sea cucumbers in all their varied beauty, both dried (top) and fresh. The dried creatures, ranging in length from a few inches to more than a foot (thirty (oh my!) cm), are powdered and taken in capsules or added to soups; fresh, they may be chopped for soups and stir-fries. (Photos by Martin Reeves)

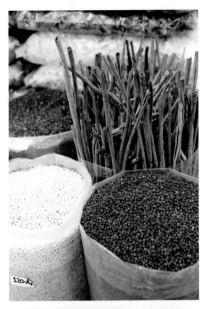
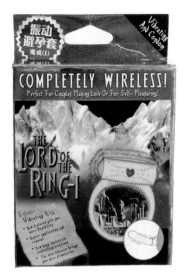
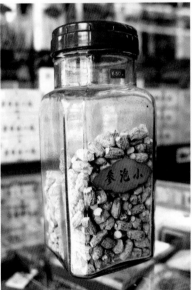
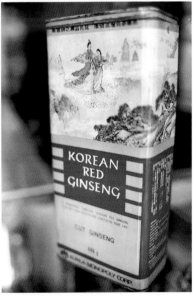

Cinnamon and white and black pepper (upper left) are among the dozens of spices regarded as sex-enhancing. A battery-operated cock ring (upper right) is slyly called The Lord of the Ring-I. Dried ginseng, Asia's most popular aphrodisiac, is shown in an apothecary jar and a tin from Korea (below). (Photos by Martin Reeves)

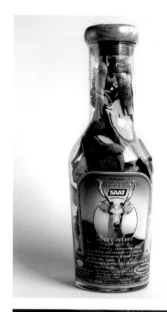
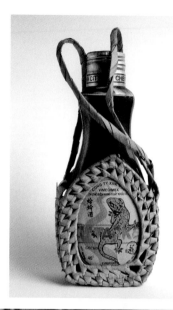
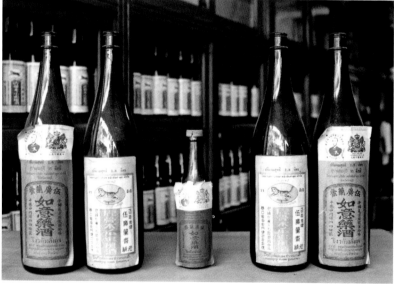

The gray slivers at the top of the bottle (top left) are shavings from a Thai deer antler, below that are dried herbs and woods to which rice wine is added and allowed to soak for a few days. The bottle top right from Vietnam contains a six-inch gecko and the bottles below from China are herbal drinks that don't include tiger parts as the labels imply. (Photos by Martin Reeves)

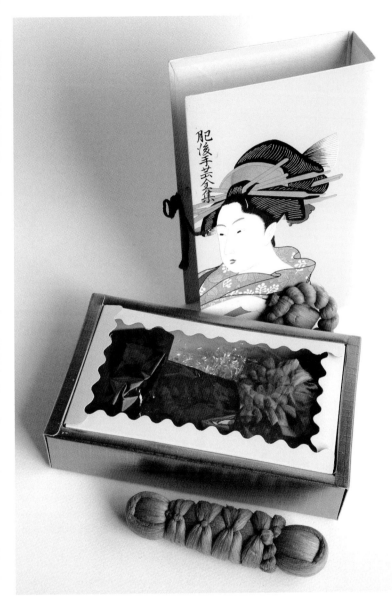

Higo *zuiki*, named for Japan's Higo province and the dried plant used to weave intricate cock rings and dildos, were distributed by the feudal lords as special gifts. The sex aids were soaked in water for several hours before use to activate chemicals in the plant that in turn stimulated those who used them. This modern copy cost $100 in the 1990s. (Photos by Martin Reeves)

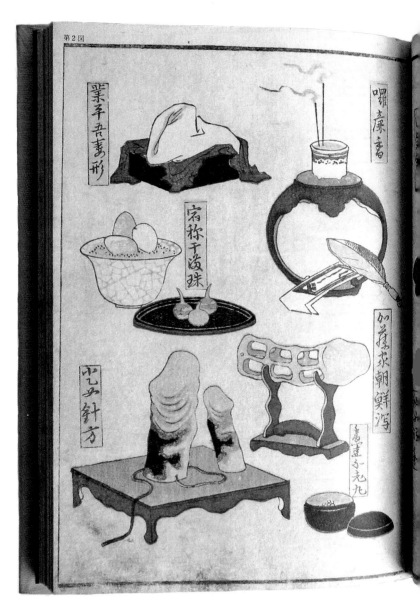

Hokusai, one of the *shunga* masters from 19th-century Japan, included depictions of sex aids as well as graphic illustrations of totally uninhibited sexual play (above and right) in wood block art that was history's first mass produced pornography, sold in thousands of retail shops. (Photos by Martin Reeves)

Fig. 2

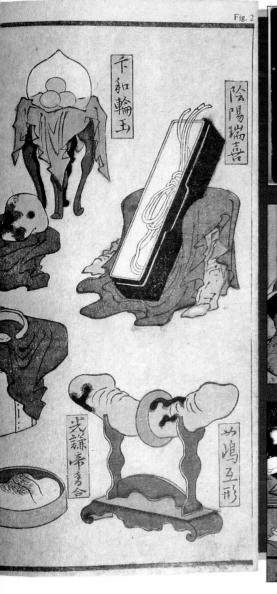

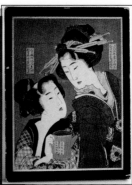

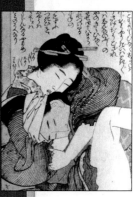

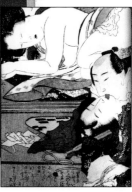

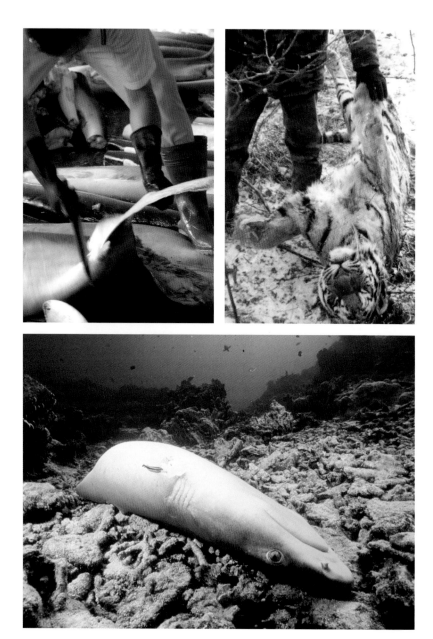

A fisherman removes a shark's fins (top left) and routinely discards the still living shark to sink to the bottom and drown or be eaten by other sharks (bottom). Tigers (top right) are treated no more respectfully. (Photos courtesy of WildAid)

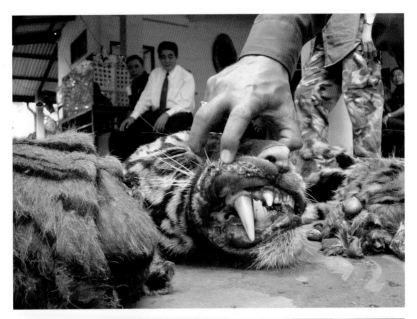

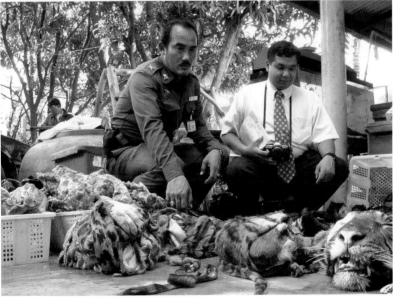

Tracking poachers in the Asian jungles nets the organization called WildAid the illegal hunters and the butchered corpses of their prey. (Photos courtesy of WildAid)

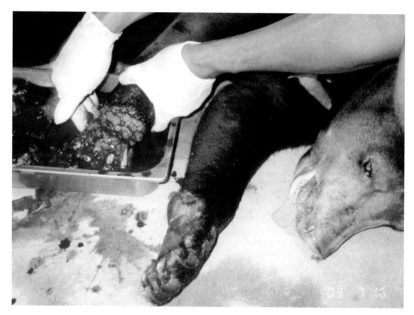

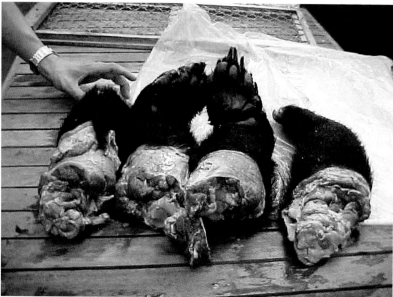

Bear paw is a treasured aphrodisiacal treat, commonly served in many parts of Asia, from China to Thailand to Indonesia, usually in a hearty stew or soup. Like tiger, this is a dish that must be ordered ahead of time. (Photos courtesy of WildAid)

animals—with a street value of $50 million.

The trade routes then led to Guangzhou in China, where Galster and a Chinese assistant, Rebecca Chen, posing as buyers, first talked with the traffickers, learning of their plan to drive the rhino to extinction. "The smugglers believed that if the rhino became extinct," Galster said, "the price of rhino horn could easily have doubled. This was a calculated attempt to corner the market using horns from one of the most valued and endangered species on earth."

Galster's sting resulted in some significant action by the Chinese authorities, including confiscation and destruction of the horn. There also was a documentary film made about the case.

In September 1993, cheers went up again in WildAid's offices when a man considered to one of Cambodia's most wanted poachers was sentenced to seven years in jail. Fifty-seven-year-old Yor Ngun was said to have tracked and killed nineteen tigers, forty leopards, thirty elephants, five hundred gaur (a species of wild cattle), and dozens of bears. WildAid had helped train some of the park rangers who, in turn, had tracked and arrested him.

This, too, was a rare occurrence. As Ben Davies said, "Never before has it been so easy or profitable to trade in wild animals, thanks to better transportation and communication links and the opening up of even the most far-flung corners of the globe. Every year, at least 25,000 primates, from two to three million birds, ten million reptile skins and more than five hundred million tropical fish are bought and sold around the world. And that's just the legal trade. The illegal smuggling of wildlife is believed to trail only the black market trade in drugs and arms."

Although progress against poaching can be seen, what

Jane Goodall calls a wildlife "holocaust" largely goes unchecked. Most Asian countries give a low priority to conservation of nature because of inadequate infrastructure, low funding, dated equipment, and inadequate training of staff. In addition, borders are porous and corrupt, laws are poorly enforced, penalties are generally light, many of the poachers are themselves off-duty military and police, and the rewards continue to be great for everyone from the poor villager up to the international syndicates. Park rangers on the front line of the fight agree that until poverty is eliminated or until the demand for wildlife product is erased, the battle to save wildlife likely will never be won.

Chapter thirteen
Great Balls of Fire

The headline on the story said it all:

CANADA REVIVES SEAL MASSACRE
Sex Organs Sold to Aphrodisiac Trade

What could be more dramatic and gruesome than white-furred baby seals bleeding to death in a landscape of snow and ice? Such photographs had appeared year after year in the media, resulting in international protest by wildlife groups and a European Community ban on the import of sealskins. This, in turn, led the Canadian government to declare a moratorium on killing the ice-breeding harp seal in 1985. Animal lovers brought out the champagne.

Ten years later, the celebration stopped. Cod had been fished to commercial extinction in the Atlantic Ocean, putting 30,000 fishermen in eastern Canada out of work, and now, in Newfoundland in February 1995, the government told these men that the cod would not regenerate in their lifetime. And while it was proven that the scarcity of fish was due to foreign over-fishing in what traditionally had been Canadian grounds, the seal also was a prodigious consumer of cod. Unable to kill European fishermen, that left the seal a handy target of opportunity, as well as a new revenue source.

A quota for what was called a "recreational" seal hunt was set at 194,000 animals, a number that was said would not endanger the species. However, because the most valued pelts came from the newborn pups, the hunt came during the birthing season when the normally nomadic seals gathered in huge numbers in a relatively small area. Death usually came by club, so as not to damage the fur.

"It's going to be bloody," said Paul Watson of the Sea Shepherd Conservation Society. "I was there the last time this happened. Every Tom, Dick, and Harry from the villages was down there trying to club seals and not doing it right and ending up skinning them alive. It'll be worse this year because they're angry [about the loss of cod]."

And so it was, and once more for five years the photographs of bloodied seal pups were published, again causing international protest. The Seal Conservation Society said, "Animal welfare violations during the hunt have been documented by conservation groups, video evidence showing seals being skinned, cut open, and dragged with hooks while still alive, being clubbed with wooden sticks or boat hooks, and being left to suffer injured for long periods before being killed. Video footage has also shown a Canadian Coast Guard ice-breaker squashing seals in its path in its efforts to give the sealers better access to the ice floes."

Why would the Canadian government risk another round of international criticism? It was politics, of course. Newfoundland, New Brunswick, Nova Scotia, and Prince Edward Island elected only a handful of representatives to

Parliament because of the small population in those provinces. Those politicians held disproportionate influence, however—in much the same way a U.S. Senator from Montana has the same vote as one from New York or California—and they represented a threat that Quebec, the fifth sealing province, might secede. This, in turn, would not only isolate the Atlantic provinces from the rest of the country, but also give them the balance of power in a perennial three-way struggle between Quebec, industrialized Ontario, and the largely agrarian west. So the fishermen-turned-sealers had to be pacified.*

By now the hunters—in Canada and Greenland and Scandinavia—had learned that the true value in bopping one of those cute little pups on the head was in the growing demand for penises in Asia. As noted by *Animal People* magazine (in which the headline above appeared), before Canada discovered the genital trade, the annual hunt averaged about 25,000 animals. Two years later, in 1997, the "Total Allowable Catch" was set at 175,000. In April 2004, before the final tally was in, it was expected that the season's kill could go as high as 350,000.

"The whole carcasses are sold and used, which enables the Canadian government to deny that the seals are being killed just for genitals," said *Animal People*. "But the genitals alone fetch up to $130 per set on the current retail market, while the pelt, meat, and oil of the seal go for about $20."

---

* In Norway in 2004, seals were blamed not only for devastating cod and other fish stocks, but also for infecting other marine life with parasites. When the private sector proposed that the annual hunt be opened to "adventure tourists"—who were "bored with survival weekends, trekking trips in the Antarctic, and booking space flights with Richard Branson," as one newspaper story put it—the Norwegian government stepped in and said no to the travel agencies but permitted the cull to continue.

And why was that? What we're talking about here is some-times called "organotherapy," referring to the belief that con-suming a healthy animal's organ will correct some ailment in the corresponding human organ. In China, the word for the practice is *jinbu*, meaning, literally, "you are what you eat."

With an estimated five to seven million thought to be in eastern Canada and another 300,000 in Greenland, the harp seal was not an endangered creature, so no efforts to intro-duce a new ban were expected.

The same could not be said for several other species, most remarkably, and tragically, the tiger. One hundred years ago, it was thought there were a hundred thousand tigers in the wild; in 2005, the total for the five existing species—the Bengal, Indo-Chinese, Siberian, South China, and Suma-tran—was down to between five and seven thousand. Another three species, the Caspian, Javan, and Balinese, had become extinct since the 1950s.

This big cat—whose dwindling numbers are still found in India, Bangladesh, Nepal, Burma, Malaysia, Thailand, Vietnam, and in the northeastern corners of Russia and China and as far south as the island of Sumatra—is killed pri-marily for its hide and bones and teeth, the skins going mainly to the Middle East where they end up on the floors and walls of men with more ego and money than good sense, the rest going to China to be ground up and sold as medicine and soup.

The tiger is killed mainly for its bones and teeth, which when powdered and taken in capsule form is believed to give those who can afford to consume it the tiger's strength, along with the status that goes with being able to afford it. This is true not just of the bone, but the genitalia. Tiger penis is famous for being sold in a soup. And, as was true with the rhinoceros, it's the animal's sexual prowess that

Asian men wished to emulate.

I defer again to my friend at the London Zoo, who told me, "Big cats—including of course tigers—mate 'briefly but continuously,' according to our most senior cat-keeper. Copulation lasts for fifteen to twenty seconds, typically recurs every twenty minutes, and will continue, day and night, for an average of four days." And since all animal penises are thought to bring strength to the lagging male human libido, what better penis to cook than that of the beast at the top of the Orient's food chain?

And so it goes all around Asia, with the cost of the real thrill and imagined benefit ranging widely, depending on which creature's penis is being chewed or sipped. In 1995, *The Atlantic Monthly* reported that $20,000 bought tiger penis soup for a dinner party of fifteen in Taiwan. (A figure I question. I've never heard a price higher than $350 per bowl, but maybe this meal also included other endangered species in the sort of banquet that is unusual but not unheard of amongst the very rich.) At the opposite end of the scale, I drank several glasses of Five Penis & Testes Wine in Guangzhou, China—where floating in the dark, fermented rice drink was a sediment purported to be the ground up genitalia of the unendangered ox, sheep, deer, dog, and snake. The price of a half liter was under $15.

Once again, all of the evidence concerning the consumption of genitals was anecdotal rather than clinical. What's more, much of the tiger penis wasn't even tiger penis. Several years ago in northern Thailand, while visiting a hill tribe village that had begun to attract tourists from China in significant numbers, I saw what were purported to be dried tiger penises for sale in one of the shops alongside the parking lot where all the buses lined up. I looked at it and when I asked the price and was told $30, I knew I was looking at a fake.

This was confirmed by Dr. Schwann Tunhikorn, head of wildlife research of Thailand's Royal Forestry Department, who said he'd never seen a real tiger penis (other than those still attached to living tigers) and that most labeled as such usually had been carved from cow tendon.

No matter. Wherever you went in Asia, personal penis power was promised at restaurants and pharmacopoeias. Rooster testicles were sold by the jar in many Chinese apothecaries and the testicles of mice—mice!—became a hot item in Taiwan after previously infertile couples reportedly conceived after eating them. A chain of restaurants offering snake and monkey and bat in Jakarta and Bali also sold packages that contained about a hundred dried snake penises for $250. (Imagine dried worms under an inch in length.) Before the onslaught of SARS led to a rewrite of the menu, eliminating much of the wildlife on it, the Imperial Herbal restaurant in Singapore across the street from the Raffles Hotel served Bull Pizzles with Chinese Yam, the cost of an entrée starting at $20 and increasing according to the number of pizzles. The restaurant also offered a selection of wines where the ingredients included deer penis, starting at $12 a glass. Not far away in the same city, I also saw a sign advertising bull penis soup for $6 and turtle penis soup for about double that, but they were all sold out.

"Chinese New Year," I was told.

Chapter fourteen
Garden Snakes & Trouser Snakes

I was in Jakarta on a magazine assignment and was joined some nights by the editor, a good friend. I was also researching a book called *Strange Foods* at that time and Tom said he'd heard that the Istana Raja Kobra in Chinatown had monkey on the menu. Upon arriving, we were told that the supply had run out. Would we settle for some fresh cobra?

I said I thought grilled or sautéed snake would be wonderful and moved toward a table. Tom said he had never eaten snake before.

"So," I suggested, "let's begin with beer."

Two bottles were brought and then our server disappeared for about ten minutes. Finally, a young man appeared, wearing shorts and a ratty tee-shirt, looking as if he'd been rousted from bed.

"Eat cobra?" he asked. We said yes. He left our table and headed toward the rear of the restaurant, beckoning us to follow. In a smaller room, about the size of a walk-in closet, one wall was floor-to-ceiling cages containing dozens and dozens of snakes that appeared to be even sleepier than our host.

The young man asked us which one we wanted. Tom noticed a bandage on the guy's hand and asked if he'd been bitten. He shrugged as if to say it happened all the time.

I pointed to one of the snakes, our guy opened the cage and approached the snake holding a metal tube under a yard (meter) long in his hands, a stiff rope passing through it, a noose at the furthest end. The idea was to catch the snake's head in the noose and pull tight at the other end of the tube, capturing it. Success! The young man then swiftly beheaded and skinned the snake by pulling it inside out, putting the skin aside for sale to a company that made wallets and belts. He then took the still-wriggling serpent to the kitchen. We returned to our table.

"Jesus," Tom said, "did you see his bandage?" I said I did. We drank some more of our beer. In a few minutes, our snake charmer returned, carrying two small glasses, each containing about an inch of warm blood. These he set before us, adding a large splash of rice wine to each, then returned to the kitchen—reappearing a moment later with a small dish containing the snake's gall bladder.

Who, he signaled, wanted it? Tom already had informed me that he was being a good sport about all this, so there was no delay in his pointing at me. The bladder, smaller than the last joint of my smallest finger, was dropped into my glass and with a nod from the snake wrangler, I lifted it and swallowed it in a single gulp. Tom did the same with his glass.

Followed very quickly on both sides of the table by more beer.

"Too bad a snake doesn't have two gall bladders," I said.

My friend shook his head and laughed. "Yeah, right. I can't tell you how disappointed I am."

Of all the creatures on the planet believed to be an aphrodisiac, the snake may be the one that gets consumed in the
greatest number, as a food or in a drink, especially in the
winter months when it is regarded by ethnic Chinese as a
"warming" food, when it feeds the needy *yang*. In Wuzhou,
Gangxi, in southwestern China, there is a snake repository
through which pass more than a million snakes a year on
their way to kitchens in Hong Kong and Macau and abroad,
wherever there is a large Chinese population.

Just outside Hanoi, there is entire village packed with
restaurants that serve exotic animals. Almost hidden away
behind a highway of garages and grocery stores about five
kilometers north of the capital, in a spot on the road called
Le Mat, snake is the dish of the day and the many restaurants
serving *thit ran* literally chase after your taxi, competing for
your palate and purse. At one of them, I was assured, "It's
very good for man." Should I not have understood, he flexed
a bicep and pointed to his groin.

Snake Alley (Huahsi Street) in Taipei, cleaned up by the
government since my first visit in the 1980s—to make it
more "suitable" for tourists, as an official website put it—in
2005 still offered the slithery creatures that gave the place its
name. Once a dark and somewhat sleazy marketplace for
stolen and counterfeit merchandise, now it was lit with an
arch of festive lights at its mouth, stretching for six or seven
reasonably tidy blocks. The open-fronted brothels on the
side streets were gone, but men still pulled snakes from wire
cages and sliced them from here to there, catching their
blood in glasses for consumption on the spot. Like carnival
barkers, speaking through wireless microphones, men in
shirtsleeves offered glasses of warm blood with pills the size
of grapes.

The sell was softer in Guangzhou, China, where I've had most of my experience eating snake. (Except, I should add, at home in rural Thailand, where my wife kills a big snake about once a month in one of her vegetable gardens and serves it later the same day, usually in a soup with ginger and lemongrass.) My favorite was the improbably named Snake King Completely and Restaurant, where I was offered a choice of seventy-five different snake dishes and seventeen snake wines.

In the gem mining town of Pailin, Cambodia, last stronghold for the Khmer Rouge, there was a woman who claimed, "I cooked cobra for Pol Pot," and up until 2000, anyway, she was still serving the dish in a small restaurant there.

In Indonesia a couple of years ago, soldiers reportedly were fed warm snake blood during an intensive six-month jungle survival course.

In Asia, you are never far from snake.

The gall bladder is said to clear the throat and lungs; the skin is ground into a paste and used as a shampoo or rubbed into the skin and scalp to combat dandruff and dermatitis. Its skin is also used to make handbags, wallets, belts, neckties, shoes, vests, and belts.

Once again, the likely reason for thinking snake has penis power is its appearance and the "law of similarity." Whatever the reason for believing the meat, blood, and organs are aphrodisiacs, however flimsy the scientific support, the demand is always there, leading to a trafficking of the reptiles that has pushed several species of cobra and other vipers onto the endangered lists. So common are the stories in the Asian newspapers they aren't considered big news, even when reporting seizures of as many as seven thousand snakes in a single raid. A story in the *Bangkok Post* reporting that many serpents confiscated from a single truck headed toward the China border not long ago was buried on one of the inside pages.

Imagine how the media in the U.S. would cover a story about seven thousand rattlesnakes being found in a truck on its way from Texas to Canada.

Chapter fifteen
Sex from the Sea

If results could be counted in headlines, the campaign to get Asians to stop eating shark fin soup was a great success. Back in 2001, when WildAid, a non-governmental organization mentioned earlier in this book in connection to its campaigns against rhino and tiger poaching, said there were dangerous levels of mercury in the fins, the claim was shouted round the world in big typeface:

> *The dangers that lurk in your bowl*
> *High mercury levels found*
> FDA *admits shark fin threat*

In Bangkok, where I live—and have eaten shark fin soup; only once and I'll explain why in a minute—fifteen of forty-five Chinatown samples were found to have more heavy metal than was considered safe.

Those restaurant owners didn't take this lightly. They filed a lawsuit against WildAid, asking $2.5 million in damages, charging the organization with distorting facts about the contamination, resulting in public confusion and misunderstanding, and consequently a loss of business.

WildAid responded by expanding its campaign to charge the shark fin industry with cruelty, exposing a practice known as "finning." This is when the sharks are pulled aboard the fishing boats, the fins are cut off, and the still living fish is then tossed back into the sea to die slowly or to be eaten by other sharks. Shark meat is, in fact, a worthy fish for anyone's menu—I've eaten it many times and it is sometimes what shows up in some parts of the world as the protein in "fish and chips"—but numerous on-board steps must be taken upon catching them to keep them safe to eat. The meat is also low-priced, but the fins are where the big money is, because it is considered a prime aphrodisiac—a claim that has never been tested or proved and on the surface seems somewhat ridiculous, putting it right up (or down) there with rhino horn and tiger penis.

The market is almost exclusively Chinese and it is a market that has exploded in the past two decades. In the old days of Maoist austerity, the official Chinese attitude was that shark fin soup was an unacceptable symbol of wealth and privilege. So from the Communist takeover in 1949, China was a relatively small player in the international trade in shark fins. That turned around in 1987 when rapid economic development, especially in southern China and Beijing, led to a big increase in disposable income and the creation of a new middle class (currently estimated at 250 million). Under Premier Deng Xiaoping, greed was suddenly good and the new affluence could now be flaunted by serving shark fin soup during Chinese New Year celebrations and at weddings, birthdays, banquets, and business meetings.

There was also the issue of "face," the obligatory respect paid to friends and associates, an important part of Chinese culture. If a businessman didn't include shark fin soup on the menu at important dinners, the host looked like a "Cheap Charlie" and, as a consequence, he lost face, as did his guests.

So what does all this have to do with improving sex? Like so much of what is considered Chinese, what is consumed at the dinner table crosses over from the traditional to the nutritional to the medicinal somewhat matter-of-factly. Just as shark fin soup will make you strong socially and impress your business colleagues, it is believed this creature whose ancestors pre-date the dinosaurs by a hundred million years also will make you a big shot in bed.

The truth is, once the complex preparation of the fins is complete—a process that takes days!—there is nothing of nutritional value left, and that's why ham and numerous other ingredients are added, to give the soup some taste. For this, depending on the amount of slippery fin in the recipe, a bowl can cost as much as $100.

"And there is your explanation," said William Schaedla of WildAid. "Those who consume it figure something that expensive must do everything it's supposed to do."

By the way, WildAid won the lawsuit and as a result of all the publicity, Thai Airways and Disney World in Hong Kong took the soup off their menus. Nonetheless, the market for fins continued to rise and showed no signs of retreating. As WildAid put it, "Sharks are likely to be in the first round of marine extinctions caused by human activity."

Aphrodite, Greek goddess of sexual intercourse, for whom aphrodisiacs are named, emerged from the sea, so it's not a bit surprising that many other waterborne creatures, like the shark, are regarded as something that will give the Asian male what he wants.*

Three of the most popular are the sea cucumber, the sea–horse, and *fugu*, the latter being a blowfish popular in Japan that will, if you get so much as a taste of its poisonous parts, make you stiff all over.

The sea cucumber, so called for its long, thick phallic shape, is one of the stranger creatures in Aphrodite's cookbook. Its movements are sluggish—it has also been called a "sea slug"—and it remains on the sea bottom from birth to death as it sucks up modest nourishment from the sediment. Related to the starfish (a species that can regenerate an arm if lost), if severely disturbed, the sea cucumber can expel its entire gastrointestinal system and within a few weeks grow a new one. At one end is its mouth, at the other its anus, which often houses a parasite in the form of a small fish which backs into the hole and lives there, feeding itself by nibbling at the host's gonads. (I'm quoting *The Oxford Companion to Food*, the definitive encyclopedia of gastronomy, here.) Is this something you'd put on your plate or in a bowl of soup?

They are found around the world, but only a few species are used as food and only in some regions, notably Asia, where the principal markets are Hong Kong, Japan, South Korea, Singapore, and Malaysia. Step on one of them in the

---

* The painter Botticelli was incorrect. She did not ride ashore on a seashell, but, according to *Hesiod's Theogony*, Chronos, son of earth and heaven, castrated his father and threw his testicles into the sea and it was from the foam of his semen that Aphrodite was born. Later, she gave birth to the androgynous god Hermaphroditos (daddy was Hermes, messenger of the gods) and then from a union with Dionysus, the god of fertility and partying, she had a son named Priapus, whose penis was permanently erect. Why someone hasn't made a mini-series of all this escapes me.

tidal waters where they can be found, as I once did in Hawaii, and it ejects sticky threads, lending more credence—to some, not to me—that it resembles a penis and thus if consumed must strengthen and encourage one's own, in the way that other similarly shaped creatures are supposed to do.

They are usually gutted, boiled, smoked, and dried in the sun, then soaked again before cooking. Low in fat content, they are said to be rich in vitamins A and C, thiamine, riboflavin, niacin, calcium, iron, magnesium, and zinc, the latter usually identified with fortifying a man's sexual response. Its history in TCM dates back thousands of years and it is prescribed for such ailments as high blood pressure and muscular disorders. The Chinese put it in soups and other dishes, while in Malaysia it is powdered and made into capsules and sold as a food supplement. Thais prefer it in spicy salads.

In contrast, the seahorse is cute. Many people keep them in aquariums as pets. But it's a strange marine animal, too. Uniquely among known animals, the male carries and hatches the eggs of the young—a parenting twist that may endear the creature to feminists, but apparently also has encouraged the belief in its medicinal properties, particularly its ability to enhance male sexual potency, though I, personally, don't understand that.

Its appearance further distinguishes it. Most are small and delicate, although some grow to twenty inches (fifty centimeters) in length. All have a horse-like head and a curling tail, and they swim upright, gliding through the sea with the grace of human swimmers performing an underwater ballet. During the two- to four-week pregnancy, when the male seahorse incubates eggs deposited in his brood pouch by the female, the partners link their tails and pirouette.

The market again is mainly in China and in Chinese communities around the world. China alone is believed to consume twenty million a year, one of the reasons that the seahorse is now farmed. Another million are thought to be sold as souvenirs, as jewelry or key rings or imbedded in Lucite paperweights. Occasionally, they appear on exotic menus. No one really has any idea how many remain in the wild, but conservationists fear that pressures of over-fishing and pollution (dredging, dumping, silting, and clearing of coastal waters) may send seahorses, as one put it, "galloping into oblivion."

I bought my first seahorse at the Qingping Market in Guangzhou. Although such privately operated (capitalist) markets are found in all Chinese cities today, it was, when it opened in 1979, one of Deng Xiaoping's more radical economic experiments. In 2003, several years after my first visit to the city, this market was pinpointed as where SARS was incubated in the civet cat and first infected humans. I must say, the market doesn't appear to have been much affected by this.

For a time, most of the live animal part of the market was shut down, as the supply went underground, but in 2005, many of the creatures were back in their old cages and shoppers were happy again. When I was researching my exotic food books, this was the part of the market that attracted my attention. Now I was more interested in the aisles of tables and stalls selling herbs and wildlife dried for ready use as Chinese medicine.

Here, there were stacks of coiled snakes and flowers pressed into pancakes the size of dinner plates. There were dried lizards of every size and variety and burlap sacks full of dried herbs of every type, their odors blending and overlapping as I made my way through the clots of morning customers and tourists taking photographs. ("Lookit that, Sheila...it's a basket of goddamned scorpions!") The two seahorses I purchased were small, only three inches (eight cm) in length; I also bought a sea cucumber, an ugly gray thing eight inches (twenty cm) long and hard enough to pound nails. I was told to reduce the creatures to a coarse powder and add it to soup or into capsules (available at any pharmacy) and swallow in the morning with green tea.

Seahorse, I was assured, was good for asthma, arteriosclerosis, broken bones, kidney disorders, skin ailments, thyroid disorders, incontinence, and you-know-what. Especially you-know-what. I tried them both when I got home, in capsules. The seahorses were powdered easily in a mortar, but I had to take a heavy metal hasp to the sea cucumber. Neither one did a thing for me. Perhaps, again, they were longtime rather than instant investments.

Seahorses are now being farmed as far away from the primary marketplace as Ireland, where Seahorse Ireland Ltd. is culturing eight species for what it calls "an almost insatiable market demand." Wholesale prices vary depending on species and size, ranging up to $630 a kilogram (2.2 pounds). Other countries that trade in seahorses include Australia, Belize, Brazil, China, Dubai, Ecuador, India, Indonesia, Italy, Japan, Kuwait, Malaysia, Mexico, New Zealand, Pakistan, the Philippines, Singapore, Spain, Sri Lanka, Tanzania, Taiwan, Thailand, the United Arab Emirates, the U.S., and Vietnam.

At last, we come to *fugu*, the Japanese blowfish with the deadly poison for which there are no antidotes, but, tragically, many anecdotes.

The consumption of flesh as dangerous as that of this puffer fish is made possible only by the extremely precise knife work of a skilled chef who must be trained, tested, and licensed before he is turned loose in a commercial kitchen. Because the poison contained in the fish's organs is far deadlier than cyanide and takes at least a dozen lives every year, including, some time ago, one of Japan's most famous *kabuki* actors, there are thirty steps in its preparation required by law, taking up to twenty minutes, compared to less than a minute to clean and fillet other species.

The gills, the sex organs, lungs, heart, gall bladder, liver, and intestines are carefully put aside and the remaining flesh is thoroughly washed to remove all trace of blood before it is boned and sliced so thinly the diner can see the pattern on the plate on which the meat is artistically arranged. This is *fugu sashimi*, the most popular way to eat it. Fins and head may be cooked separately with other ingredients or the entire fish can be battered and fried.

The *kabuki* star, Mitsugora Bando, was not the only well known person poisoned by this fish. The explorer Captain James Cook and the fictional spy James Bond were only made seriously ill. I was not with Michael Freeman, who took the photographs for my books *Strange Foods* and *Extreme Cuisine*, so I did not have the opportunity to share the meal with him. It's just as well. He told me the bill came to $1,200!

Which I guess explains why Japanese men, and others who place bravado ahead of cash, think *fugu* has aphrodisiacal powers. After spending that much on dinner—and living to tell the tale—what better way to celebrate than to race off to bed?

Chapter sixteen
Birds Do It...

One reason that a bowl of birds' nest soup is so pricey—sometimes more than $100 a bowl, depending on the quality of the nests from which it was made and the fanciness of the restaurant in which it is served—is the difficulty encountered in collecting the nests.

To begin with, the locations where the nests of the sea swift may be found are limited to remote seaside areas in southern Thailand, Malaysia, and Borneo (a part of Malaysia), where over hundreds of thousands of years, erosion and other geological forces carved out one of the largest, most intricate cave systems in the world. Long abandoned by human inhabitants, Borneo's caves support unusual forms of life, among them the small swifts who build nests on the walls of these deep, dark caves using their spittle. These small, half-teacup sized nests that may take up to two months of work, may be more than three hundred feet (a hundred meters) up a sheer cliff and must be harvested in the dark.

To reach the nests, collectors construct precarious bamboo ladders, many of which are no more than poles lashed together with vine, then climb the wobbly contraptions holding in one hand "four-branched, spear-like implements—fixed to a handle several yards in length—and provided at the top with a lighted candle end. Holding fast with his left hand to the ladder, he gives the nest a poke with his long tool and loosens it from its support, then hauls it down, takes it off the spiked fork and lays it in a rattan basket fastened around his waist." (I'm quoting here from a 1928 account, but little has changed.) It is no surprise that many of the collectors fall to their deaths every year in the process.

There are further risks. Because these small nests generally are found on public land, the rights to collect are regulated by the Malaysian and Thai governments and assigned by area, for which the commercial harvesters pay millions of dollars in fees. Poachers are attracted, some of them led by moonlighting employees, and guards with automatic weapons are told: shoot to kill. Many die every year, some of whom are found with magic amulets in their mouths that were thought to protect them from such an ugly end.

Another reason a bowl of soup costs so much is the extraordinarily long preparation time. Although dried nests are sold to home cooks in Asian groceries and Chinese herbal shops—priced in the hundreds of dollars for a package that may weigh no more than a large handful of popcorn—most of the soup is consumed in restaurants because of the hours-long effort required for soaking, rinsing, and simmering.

The status attached to eating the soup is a third reason. Take the boss out to dinner, put it on the menu for a special event such as a birthday or a wedding, and you look like a Big Spender, a Generous Guy.

So what does the Big Spender get for his money? Not much. The nests and the dishes made from them have been studied extensively and shown to be high in water-soluble protein, as much as sixty per cent of volume, and that could promote cell division in the immune system, which is good. But it's also been made clear that all but a tiny part of one per cent of that protein is removed by the complex preparation, along with whatever taste the nest had to begin with. The Nutrition Research Institute at Mahidol University in Thailand said twenty-six bottles of a popular birds' nest drink together costing about $100 offered the protein found in one egg.

No one knows exactly how long birds' nest has been regarded as a Chinese delicacy. Academics say at least 1,500 years, although reliable documentation goes back only to the eighteenth century. What is certain is the value, with the most translucent and least contaminated of the nests selling for as much as $2,000 per kilogram. No wonder that, like the tiger penis, counterfeit birds' nests command a part of the market.

So far, there is no proof of any aphrodisiacal effect.

A more commonly consumed product than the nest of the bird is the egg, and in Asia, the one that makes it onto the aphrodisiacs list is the fertilized egg of the duck with a partially developed embryo inside that is boiled and eaten from the shell. It is most popular in the Philippines, where it is called *balut*, but also is sold widely in Vietnam (and called *ho bit long*) and to smaller markets in China (where it is thought to have originated and today is called *maodan*) and in Laos, Cambodia, Thailand, Malaysia, and Indonesia, as well as in cities elsewhere in the world where there is a sizeable Chinese, Filipino, or Vietnamese population.

High-tech processing of the eggs has come slowly to the Philippines, both the producers and consumers believing that the traditional way is best. Thus, most of the hundreds of thousands sent to the marketplace every week in Manila alone are incubated in burlap sacks that are sunk into long, rectangular boxes filled with rice husks, the bags of eggs further insulated by a burlap bag filled with more husks placed on top. The result is a reasonable simulation of the temperature that would have been provided by mama duck, 42.5°C or 108°F.

If full incubation were permitted, the eggs would hatch in twenty-eight days. Testing begins at six days and those found to be infertile are cured in salt, dyed red so they won't be confused with fresh eggs, and taken straight to the shops. On the fourteenth day, the remaining eggs are held in front of a light again and if the shadow revealed indicates the embryo hasn't developed properly, these eggs are boiled and called *penoy*. They look, smell, and taste much like a normal hard-boiled egg, but you can tell that there's something happening, bird-wise.

What are called *balut* are those removed on the seventeenth or eighteenth day and shown on the third examination to contain a healthy, living embryo. These, too, are boiled and along with the *penoy* are rushed to the city streets where vendors keep them warm in buckets of sand or insulated baskets, crying out "*Penoy...balut!*" They sell with small packets of salt for about twenty-five U.S. cents apiece, in the morning as a daily lift-off, in the evening as an aphrodisiac, to be consumed at home, often taken with beer or gin.

Balut are usually eaten with a bit of salt, the larger or flatter end of the egg held upwards and opened carefully until a small, coin-sized hole reveals a thin white tissue covering. This is removed, the salt is added, and the liquid is sipped like a broth. The eggshell is then further removed and eaten as any hard-boiled egg, with more salt added to taste; some also add a few drops of vinegar or a bit of chili. The entire egg is consumed except for the hard knot of egg white at the bottom, which won't do any harm if eaten but usually is discarded.

At seventeen days, the egg is said to be *balut sa puti* ("wrapped in white") and the embryo inside isn't old enough to show its beak, feathers, bones, or feet. This is the preferred "age" in the Philippines. In Vietnam, most eggs are marketed from nineteen to twenty-one days into the incubation period, when the chick is old enough to be recognizable as a baby duck, its skeleton firm but tender when cooked.

As a snack, its fans say it can't be beat—for its combination of saltiness and sweetness, its softness and crunchiness, its tartness and stickiness. Nowadays, in this age of anything-goes cuisine, in nouvelle whatever restaurants, *balut* is also oven-baked, deep-fried, cooked in a pastry, or included in a bisque.

As for its value as an aphrodisiac, however, again there is no, ahem, hard evidence.

Both eggs and cooked birds have been credited with such power, nonetheless. "Have sex as often as possible," advised *The Golden Lotus*, one of the early Chinese guidance love scrolls. "Eat the products of flying birds such as sparrows' eggs and rooster meat. Rooster meat contains male hormones. If you eat it, your 'jade wand' will become erect once more. When it is erect, it is ready and willing to perform the 'opening of the jade stone.' When it is completely aroused, get started.

"Encourage it by eating sparrows' eggs. However, if your erection is not hard enough, marinate the sparrows' eggs in wheat porridge or in malt. It you eat it, your impotence will disappear.

"This is Danchang's method for curing impotence by

swallowing the life force of birds."

And then there is McQueen's bustard. Hunting this bird has been illegal since 1972 in Pakistan, one of the few places where it may still be found, unless you are one of the Pakistani government's honored guests and invest in its development. Mary Ann Weaver wrote in the *New Yorker* that most of these guests came from the Middle East, where the bird had been hunted to extinction.

"Many Pakistanis are puzzled by the royal hunts, and can't really explain why, with the arrival of the *hobara*, scores of Middle Eastern potentates—presidents, ambassadors, ministers, generals, governors—descend upon their country in fleets of private planes," she wrote. "They come armed with computers and radar, hundreds of servants and other staff, customized weapons, and priceless falcons, which are used to hunt the bird."

More birds have gone into the cook pot in India, where bird-catching is an ancient art that once was handed down from father to son. There, not so long ago, sparrows were captured when large nets were thrown over trees where the birds came to roost; the catch sometimes numbered in the thousands.

Once more, the proof was not in the pudding.

Chapter seventeen
Bees Do It…

I was having a drink with a friend in a Bangkok bar not far from where he and I both live and we were talking about this book when he asked if I were including bee pollen.

"Bee pollen," I said. It was more a statement than a question. I knew about bee pollen and tended to regard it as one of those New Age substances that was supposed to cure just about everything, and was hugely overpriced, and now I said as much.

My friend said, "Oh, no, you have it wrong." He then told me about meeting an older woman in Hat Yai in the south of Thailand some time earlier who sold him a bottle of the golden granules, telling him it would make him "strong." As she did so, my friend said, she flexed an arm and made a fist and threw a look somewhere between his belt and his knees. He tried it and said he now swore by it, had just bought a kilogram of the stuff.

A book I had come to regard as an essential source on the subject of aphrodisiacs (however over enthusiastic and accepting its author often seemed), Christian Räatsch's *Plants of Love*, had an entire chapter about honey and other bee products, but the emphasis was on the medieval drink called mead and most of his references (as is so often the case in the literature of aphrodisiacs) came from the Christian Bible's Old Testament, the ancient Greeks and Romans, and such. I was writing a book about Asia, so I didn't give Räatsch much attention initially when he so lavishly praised the bee.

After talking with my friend, I went through my library again, and logged onto the Internet for a further search, and headed off to a shop where "food supplements" played a significant role in the product line, realizing sooner than I wish to admit that I had overlooked the obvious. Honey and other bee product was so pervasive in its use in the world of aphrodisia, I hadn't noticed its presence, I had come to think of it in the same way "just add water" appears on packages of instant noodle soups. Clearly, I hadn't given the buzzing bee the importance it deserved.

I don't know why I was so blind. Hadn't I recently encountered bottles of honey spiked with ginger in Jakarta when I was exploring *jamu*—the honey used to soften the bitterness of many of the herbs, but also, perhaps, to add something on its own? How about the time my daughter and I returned to Sapa, Vietnam, after a day of trekking the tribal villages and being told that the best thing for renewed energy was bee wine (bees fermented in rice wine)?

Hadn't I also recorded its use as an ingredient in recipes from the *Kama Sutra* and other early Indian and Chinese texts? A fourteenth-century explorer named Ibn Battuta praised the aphrodisiac properties of honey saying, "Ten days after we had embarked from Calcutta, we safely reached the island of Dibat-el-Halal. It lies in the midst of numerous other islands, all of which are occupied by upright Moslems. Using honey and coconut, they prepare a type of mead that, in combination with certain fish that are their primary sustenance, bestows upon them a virility unlike any that can be found in any other people. The inhabitants of this island are capable of amazing things with their wives, but even I, a stranger, was blessed with these powers. As long as I stayed on the island, I had four rightful women, and was ready for them every day, yet I also visited whichever one of my concubines whose turn it happened to be—and this for eighteen months."

Most important, I'd overlooked what the bee was doing: fertilizing! It was conveying the fertilizing element of flowering plants, consisting of fine, powdery yellowish grains, from one blossom to the next, *ad* practically *infinitum*. The bee was, thus, in an anthropomorphic way, having "sex" thousands of times a day! What a revelation that was. (If somewhat delusional.)

Dictionary definition: honey is the sweet, viscous substance made from nectar gathered from flowers by the common honey bee, *Apis mellifera* and *A. dorsata*, insects that preceded humans on earth by ten to twenty million years. Honeybees are one of the oldest forms of animal life and honeycombs of wild bees were the only available sweet as far back as 7000 BC. It is made up of sugars—fructose, glucose, maltose, and sucrose; no surprise, then, that it's regarded as a quick source of human energy. Honey is also rich in minerals, amino acids, enzymes, and B-complex vitamins. So it's also said to be good for whatever ails you.

Aside: mead, a word that derives from the Sanskrit word for honey, *madhu*, is believed to have been the world's first intoxicating drink.

Honey isn't easy to produce. One hundred and sixty thousand bees make trips to some two million flowers to gather the four pounds of nectar it takes to make one pound of honey. Estimates of energy consumption indicate that foraging bees fly more than seven million flight miles (eleven million kilometers) for every gallon (four liters) of honey. All this effort and the most any individual bee will make in a lifetime will equal about one teaspoon. Think about this the next time you put a jar of the stuff in your shopping cart.

The flavor and color of honey are highly variable, depending on the flowers visited by the bees while making their workaholic rounds. The taste and scent thus change according to which fruit, which herb, which scented tree predominate; this is one of Mother Nature's gentlest and most loving acts of fertilization (sex), shared by a number of birds and butterflies. The honey may be further flavored by the addition of herbs and other ingredients before sealing the bottle, as was the case in Jakarta, where ginger was added for oomph.

Honey isn't the only bee product. About ten years ago, I attended one of those high-pressure, New Age sales presentations in a Bangkok hotel where the object was to create a pyramidal sales force to sell bee pollen. Most of the people in the audience were women—virtually all of them Thai, as was the friend I accompanied—and although I didn't understand all the woman on stage was saying, she was mesmeric. She praised bee pollen and read from what she said were medical reports, spinning a web (hive?) of mystery and delight. She called other women to the microphone so they could tell their stories of miraculous cures and newfound strength. The latter would be of especial interest, the moderator stepped in and said, to women who wanted to rekindle dwindling passion in their men. Put a little of the stuff in his rice soup in the morning, a little more in his stir-fry at night, and watch out!

My friend said she was thinking about signing up and we met with a Thai man after the meeting, one of the people I knew were there to "close" the sale, adding more pigeons to the pyramid. All I really remember of the encounter is the size of the diamond in his pinky ring—a symbol of the program's bottom line appeal to greed: get in early and sign up ten of your friends, each of whom will sign up ten more, and so on, all of whom share their profits with you, and you'll be sitting on top of a fortune! I'm happy to report that my friend didn't go along.

Honey is the most popular bee product, likely because it is the most affordable, and pollen may be No. 2. This is the male seed of flowers that is transported from flower to flower by the bee, a portion of the microscopic golden dust falling off the bee's body with each visit to pick up more. According to a webpage that sold the stuff, each bee pollen pellet contained "over two million flower pollen grains and one teaspoonful contained over two and a half billion grains." No wonder it costs so damned much.

But it is rich in proteins (about forty per cent is protein), free amino acids, vitamins including B-complex, and folic acid, aiding recovery from chronic illness, adding weight during convalescence, reducing cravings, regulating the intestines, building new blood, preventing infectious diseases such as the cold and flu (it had antibiotic type properties), and helping overcome retardation and other developmental disorders, not to mention contribute all that bedtime bounce.

It would seem presumptuous to complain.

More Buzz

The bee is not the only insect in the aphrodisiac inventory. In fact, one of the most praised is a creature called "Spanish Fly"—which is not a fly at all, but a small beetle, *Lytta vesicatoria*, somewhat more commonly known as *cantharides*. This is not Asian—it's African—and I won't dwell on it, except to say that it was not unknown in ancient China, where it was made up in the form of electuaries containing honey, saffron, cinnamon, nutmeg, cloves, and cubeb peppers.

More recently it reached Asian shores again. In December 2005, Thailand's Food and Drug Administration warned of potential lethal side effects when it was reported being consumed by teenagers in Chiang Mai. It's apparently true, though rare, that its consumption can be risky and possibly fatal if you take too much of the dried and powdered creature, but no one—no one!—questions its effectiveness. In the world of Mother Nature's aphrodisiacs, this is at or near the top of almost everyone's Oh boy! list.

There are other insects, too. In an earlier chapter, the use of "the bristles of certain insects that live in trees" (unidentified as to species) to enlarge a man's *lingam* was advised in the *Kama Sutra*. In a silk-sheet manuscript found more than two thousand years ago in a Chinese tomb, assigned the title "*Yangsheng fang*" ("Recipes for nurturing life"), it was suggested that a chicken be plucked and hung alive on a pole and then rubbed against several bee hives until it died from the stings; its flesh was then finely pounded, mixed with other ingredients to make a paste, and daubed on cloth napkins, which then were applied to the man's feet. In a second recipe, a napkin soaked in a liquid containing red ants, blister beetles, and a third stinging insect (again unidentified) was used prior to intercourse: "rub the jade whip [penis] with it and the horse [vagina] will then be startled."

For those who may think I condescend, I wish to point out that the same manuscript, found in what is called the Mawangdui tomb (burial dated to 168 BC in Hunan province), also first described the Chinese *qing hao* plant, which is the source of the most promising anti-malarial drug, artemisinin, being used by modern medicine today. In other words, don't knock it until you've tried it.

More recently in China, hornet's larvae have been used in the same way as bee larvae, cooked or raw, to ease stomach pains and serve as a sexual stimulant. So, too, hornets' and wasps' nests, incinerated, the ashes mixed with water.

Pulverized, dried cicada; horn decoctions made from the rhinoceros beetle (it had a penis-like horn, too, though very small); dried silkworm cocoons; the list of love bugs went on and on. But outside Spanish Fly, the only insect that I heard about that really worked as I was writing this book, came when a friend called to say he had been bitten by a small but ferocious scorpion, measuring about two inches (five centimeters) from pincers to barbed tail.

It happened in southeastern Thailand near the Cambodian border in the middle of the night. Jamie said he woke up screaming. Then as the pain receded and numbness followed, his penis stiffened, and it was a full day later before he and it were back to "normal." Jamie said he did not consider this a wonderful aphrodisiac event.

"It was like getting a shot of a local anesthetic," Jamie said. "We were holidaying with friends and my wife made a joke of it at the beach all day."

Chapter eighteen
Herbal Whisky, Scorpion Wine & a Serpent's Beating Heart

I was wandering the aisles with my wife at a food fair in Bangkok and came upon a booth offering deer antler, sold powdered in capsule form and thinly sliced in combination with numerous other herbs and small shavings of medicinal wood, all stuffed into a decanter, to be filled at home with rice wine and left for a while to steep.

Another time, upon entering a five-star hotel near the Laos border in northern Thailand, I noticed a bottle of rice wine behind the bar with a scorpion at the bottom.

In China, as noted elsewhere in this book, I drank a lot of what was called Five Penis & Testes Wine, containing the dried and ground genitals of dog, ox, deer, sheep, and snake.

In Vietnam, I encountered not only a variety of snakes coiled at the bottom of recycled bottles—cobra being the most popular, some of them small enough to fit into those little Johnny Walker bottles you see on airlines and in hotel mini-bars—but also a gecko so large I marveled at how they got the sucker in there.

In Laos, centipedes can show up in your glass, in China bear bile, and in Cambodia in the 1990s so many toads were being killed for their hallucinogenic oils and added to wine that the government said stop, or the bufo species would become extinct, leading to an infestation of insects; people were getting sick and dying as well, as the bufo was known to exude poisonous oils.

All over Asia, other preventive and curative ingredients went into whisky, usually a mixture of herbs. In the rural rice growing countryside in Thailand where my wife and I have a home, bits of dried bark and wood cut from trees in the area, along with berries and herbs, are soaked in a Thai type of rice "whisky" and taken by the shot to begin the day or to give the start of the evening a boost.

The literature was there, too. Christian Räatsch in *Plants of Love* offered recipes for wine spiked with mandrake root, ginger, galangal, cubeb pepper, hemp, and opium—all, individually, recognized as aphrodisiacs.

"We have found," explained Dr. Santi Watthana, a botanist at the Queen Sirikit Botanical Garden in Chiang Mai, Thailand, "that the reason whisky is used to make *yaa dong* [Thai for alcohol with herbs and other ingredients] is so that the alcohol can act as the solvent. It is a better solvent than water, and also keeps the herbs from spoiling. In addition, whisky raises the body temperature and causes the blood to circulate more quickly. When drunk in the right quantity, whisky itself is a kind of medicine."

Wine snobs criticize such libations harshly because of the high alcohol content—thirty-nine per cent in the snake wine I'm drinking as I write this, contrasted with most table wines' ten to thirteen per cent—and since most of the consumers of this viper vino are in China and Southeast Asia, where the tendency is to toss it back in one gulp (a traditional Chinese toast is "*Gambei!*" meaning "empty glass"), we who drink it are often considered barbarians. We make no attempt to test the wine's "nose" and "mouth" (wine snob talk for aroma and taste) or to judge the liquid by its viscosity and the way it was racked, aged, bottled, and corked. Our concern is: will it make us strong? Will it get us not only off, but up?

Most of the alcohol drunk in Asia doesn't contain such exotic ingredients and it is consumed for the same reasons that it's downed anywhere else, for the taste and the camaraderie that accompanies its consumption, and for the buzz or blotto that comes when swallowed in sufficient quantity. As elsewhere, it also is thought to be a sexual stimulant.

There are good reasons. First, in small quantities it depresses the brain centers that control fear, thereby reducing the individual's anxiety. More important, it often diminishes inhibitions, thereby creating a temporary increase in libido—or a way for the libido to escape the chains of caution and shyness. And as the good doctor from Chiang Mai said, it's good for the circulation and that's always good for any sexual act that may follow.

This is hardly a new idea. Alcohol and sex surely have been linked ever since the first drink was fermented. This connection has been the subject of much writing in Asia. An anonymous twelfth century Indian poet wrote about a woman named Ramaprasada:

Who is this dark beauty coming this way?
Who can she be, young and lovely,
Naked yet devoid of shame, charming everyone she meets?
See how she walks, loose-hipped—
How unseemly for such a respectable lady.
She's clearly been at the wine...

In the "Laws of Manu" from *The Sacred Books of the East*, an Indian text first translated in 1895 and reprinted in 2001, much the same story was told, but even more critically. The author, perhaps a Hindu, Muslim or Sikh (religions that forbid alcohol consumption), wrote of "women that throw off their clothes, and so dance, clouded by heady drink, that pair without heed of any barrier, and live as their lusts dictate; that piss standing, like the ass or camel, have lost decency and virtue, and in all things are without shame—the son of such as these, though would'st speak here of virtue!

"If the Madra woman is asked for sour rice gruel (an intoxicating drink), she shakes her buttocks, and utters—she who is always giving herself—these dreadful words: 'Let none ask me for my beloved sour rice gruel...'"

The writer continued: "When the women have taken a heavy drink of corn and molasses and taken cow's flesh with garlic—they, who eat cakes, flesh, and roasted barley, and know not the ways of goodness, sing and dance, drunk and unclothed on the earth-walls of the city and of the houses, without wreaths and unanointed, and amidst drunken, lewd songs of various kinds, which sound like the noise of asses and camels. They know no restraint in their pairings, and in all things they follow their lust..."

This, of course, is what a lot of men in Asia—and likely everywhere else on the planet—are looking for. This is why there are so many sex venues where alcohol is so key to the entertainment format. Karaoke bars in Japan, China, and South Korea...go-go bars across Southeast Asia...et cetera.

Such a connection goes back hundreds of years. In all the early erotic art of India, China, and Japan, the lusty members of the respective countries' aristocracy were pictured drinking at the same time they were having sex, the woman shown lifting a cup of boozy sustenance to her lover's lips as they changed positions from The Cricket's Clasp to The Deer That Lifts Its Horns.

Nicholas Bornoff in his book about Japanese sex, *Pink Samarai* (1991) wrote, "Alcohol is if anything a more frequent prelude to sex in Japan than anywhere else. Measuring only some two inches [five centimeters] across as though to beg frequent refills from a charming companion, sake cups are much given to suggestiveness. Erotic cups were brazenly decorated with copulating couples of *shunga* inspiration and during the Edo period, and in the Meiji era, they often came to be covered with lids. Although the adoption of western propriety commanded discretion, the cups were used only where they were least likely to offend—in brothels and in 'teahouses' that never served tea.*"

Today, clumsy replicas of these vessels are sold as souvenirs—in much the same way small versions of the *lingam* and *yoni* statues found in so many town squares in India are sold to foreigners, and in Thailand the *phlad kikh* (the phallic figures believed to protect the wearer from evil spirits and make him prosperous) are mass produced in a kind of plastic and hawked on the streets in tourist neighborhoods. In Japan there is also a cup that is shaped like a mushroom with a hole in the middle of the "mushroom's" head, through which the salaryman drinks.

There can be no doubt that, with rational limitations set by the drinker—man or woman—alcohol seems to work as a sexual stimulant. No one is more enthusiastic than Dan Reid, who said in his book *The Tao of Health, Sex and Longevity*, "So fundamental is alcohol to Chinese medicine, that the defining element in the written ideogram used to form the

---

* *Shunga* is early Japanese erotic art. See "From Pillow Talk to Pornography" page 221.

words 'medical' and 'doctor' is the symbol for 'wine.'"

Dan also echoed the words of the Thai doctor who said alcohol was a good host for medicinal ingredients. And he did so in presenting a very complex recipe for what the Chinese called *yao-jiou*, or "medicine wine," also known as Spring Wine: "Spring Wine is made by steeping potent medicinal herbs in strong alcoholic spirits for up to a full year, during which time the essential active elements are extracted from the herbs by the spirits. This is one of the most ancient methods on record for preparing Chinese herbal prescriptions, for Chinese physicians discovered long ago that alcohol not only extracts, absorbs and preserves the active ingredients in herbs, but also facilitates their rapid assimilation from stomach to bloodstream, and catalyzes their metabolism in the tissues to which they travel."

Dan called Spring Wine a great "appetizer" for food and sex, making the drinker hungry for both. Taken on an empty stomach, it "perks up the libido, stimulates glandular secretions, enhances blood circulation and flushes the organs with heat and energy." The list of ingredients was long and several were quite strange, but Dan said they could be found at any "genuine Chinese herb shop," not only in Asia but also in any large metropolitan Chinatown, although I ran into a wall with a couple of them; you'll recognize which ones.

In the order presented, this is his complete shopping list: deer horn shavings, deer horn resin, resin made from the hides of wild black donkeys, horny goat weed, rehmannia rhizome, astragalus root, eucommia bark, Chinese wolfberry, Japanese wax-privet seeds, cynomorium stems, dried human placenta, Korean ginseng root, raspberry seeds, seahorse, and red-spotted lizard. All were to be placed in a glass or ceramic vat of eight to ten liter capacity, with six liters of brandy, rum, or vodka added. The container was to be sealed and let sit for from three to six months. Half was then to be poured into bottles through a funnel lined with several layers of cheesecloth or gauze. Three more liters were to be added to the remaining herbal stew and left to steep for another three to six months, when the straining process was repeated, resulting in a total of nine bottles. These were to be sweetened with lumps of crystal rock sugar, honey, or fructose syrup to blunt the bitterness. Two to three ounces daily during the winter, half that during the warmer months.

"Candy is dandy," wrote Dorothy Parker, an American, "but liquor is quicker." So, too, it is in the East. However, as with all alcoholic drinks, caution is advised. Most people quote Shakespeare, who warned in *Macbeth*: "It provokes the desire, but it takes away the performance. Therefore [the Porter continued] much drink may be said to be an equivocator with lechery; it makes him, and it mars him; it sets him on, and it takes him off; it persuades him, and disheartens him; makes him stand to, and not stand to; in conclusion, equivocates him in a sleep, and, giving him the lie, leaves him."

A Japanese proverb says it as well and more succinctly: "At the first cup man drinks wine, at the second wine drinks wine, at the third wine drinks man."

Chapter nineteen
Better Loving, Through Chemistry

I was not new to dance halls and drugs. The two worked very well together back in the 1960s in America when I was writing for *Rolling Stone* magazine and large, long-unused spaces were given new life by an explosion of popular music, spreading from the Fillmore Auditoriums in San Francisco and New York to the Roundhouse (a long-disused railroad roundhouse) in London. At that time, the music was rock and roll and the drugs were mainly marijuana, hashish, and LSD, and for the more exotic trippers, peyote and mescaline, what scientists called "psychotropic" drugs and we all called "psychedelics."

Since then, the scene has changed several times but only slightly, occurring again in America with the advent of "disco music," a rock offshoot led by John Travolta and the Bee Gees in *Saturday Night Fever* (1977) and the "rave" parties in England. In time, the phenomenon spread to the capitals of Asia, as the music fractured and audiences were offered a dozen forms. By the end of the twentieth century, the most popular in the cool nightclubs and cavernous discotheques were "techno," "house," and "trance," mutant, electronic forms without lyrics or melody that seemed aimed mainly at disturbing blood pressure and pulse, accompanied by volume that led to aural distress.

The drugs had changed as well. Now, they were virtually all produced in laboratories rather than harvested from the forests and fields. All that seemed similar was the various governments declaring the new drugs as illegal as the old ones.

The drugs, also now as before, were considered to be aphrodisiacs, and the greatest of these was MDMA, chemical shorthand for 3,4-methylenedioxymethamphetamine, more commonly known as "E" or Ecstasy.

Although it was first synthesized in 1912 by the German pharmaceutical company Merck for possible use as an appetite suppressant, over half a century passed before it was tested on humans, after it was unearthed in some old and forgotten medical literature by an American scientist named Alexander Shulgin, who became known for this discovery as "Dr. Ecstasy." After testing it on himself (one of more than four thousand "trips" he said in 2005 that he had taken), he was convinced it could be used to treat mental illness and passed it along to hundreds of therapists.

Further study declared its primary effect was to stimulate the secretion of large amounts of serotonin as well as dopamine and noradrenaline in the brain [individually considered by many to be aphrodisiacs], causing a general sense of openness, empathy, energy, euphoria, and well-being. Tactile sensations were believed enhanced for some users, making general physical contact with others more pleasurable. All of which might have made it sound like a good thing to have on the shelf next to the aspirin bottle, but as it came to be used as a "recreational" drug, the Powers That Hate Fun Drugs came crashing down and in 1985 it was classified as a "Schedule 1" substance due to what the U.S. government deemed a lack of medicinal benefit and high potential for abuse.*

Making it illegal didn't halt its use at all and today, the drug that was reborn in the USA and in the 1980s was adopted by the "rave" parties of England (where "ravers" held their drug-fuelled dances in open fields and abandoned warehouses, the temporary locations spread by word of mouth), is the drug of choice for Asia's consumer generation and factories from Burma to Malaysia to southern China to Taipei to Indonesia are pumping out a ready supply.

In an effort to curb such activity, since 2003 police have raided the trendiest nightclubs in numerous Asian cities, forcing everyone present to submit to a urine test before being allowed to go home. Should the blue liquid turn purple when the urine is added, it's off to jail you go, even though it's been established that a variety of antihistamines and other prescription drugs can produce the same result as Ecstasy and amphetamines.

Ecstasy had another downside. Because it was manufactured illicitly, some tablets or capsules contained varying mixtures of MDMA and related drugs (including amphetamines) as well as other substances and impurities. Many of the candy-colored pills also proved to be fake or contained

---

* Its ability to facilitate self-examination with a reduced fear has since proved useful in some therapeutic settings, however, leading to its approval in 2001 by the FDA for testing in patients with post-traumatic stress syndrome. By 2005, it was being prescribed for American soldiers traumatized by fighting in Iraq and Afghanistan to help free them of flashbacks and recurring nightmares. It was still illegal for use by people who merely wanted to dance and fuck.

little or no MDMA. This is a problem common to all illegal drugs; when money is to be made and there is no quality control, there are consequent risks.

Ecstasy also tended to raise body temperatures, especially if large amounts of non-alcoholic liquid (water, fruit juices) weren't consumed while tripping. Tests further showed that while Ecstasy could lower sexual inhibitions, men often couldn't get erections while high. This led to taking Ecstasy with Viagra (or another of the ED pharmaceuticals), a combination sometimes called "sextasy."

Ecstasy may have been the dance crowd's favorite chemical concoction in Asia, but it wasn't alone. Even more prevalent, but less frequently connected to sex, were the amphetamines that became the overall drug of choice in much of Southeast and East Asia. Initially popularized during the Second World War when it was given to pilots and soldiers to keep them alert and somewhat crazed for more hours, it's now used by students, long distance truck drivers, and others who want to stay awake longer than Mama Nature might think wise. (It also is used to keep elephants working in illegal logging in Southeast Asia, addicting many of them.)

Law enforcement authorities—not always the most reliable of sources, as their budgets tend to rise parallel to the alarmist tendencies their reports often take—said in 2001 that illegal amphetamine manufacture seemed to be concentrated in Burma and China, but was also emerging in the Philippines, Malaysia, and Indonesia, while North Korea was reported to be a major supplier of the drug to Japan.

Though various manifestations of the hemp plant (marijuana, *ganja*, *bhang*, hashish, et cetera) continued to be the most popular drugs with reported aphrodisiac qualities in Asia, in 2005 amphetamines surely were Number Two.

Collectively known as "speed," this family of chemicals is commonly taken as an appetite suppressant. In low doses, it also has been shown to increase libido and sexual pleasure, raise blood pressure (which might deliver ancillary priapic benefit), retard ejaculation, and enhance orgasmic pleasure.

Even at moderate doses, however, impotence becomes more common in men and decreased libido occurs in both sexes. At high doses, some intravenous amphetamine users have reported what is technically known as "pharmacogenic orgasm," or drug-generated orgasm, although it has nothing to do with sexual intercourse. Amphetamines also can cause both acute and chronic toxicity. In Thailand, it's called *yaa baa*, which literally means "crazy medicine."

Sounding equally "crazy" to me is the use of Ketamine, also called "K." This is a surgical anesthetic developed in the 1960s and used on the battlefields of Vietnam. Today, it's found primarily in veterinary medicine and sparingly in humans, mostly with infants and the elderly. In street dosages—popped as a pill, snorted as a powder, or injected in liquid form—it works on the receptors in the brain that are triggered by opium, resulting in hallucinations, and for some users deep disorientation and a near catatonic state, known as the "K hole." I haven't tried it. It reminds me of Quaaludes, another heavy downer popular a couple of decades ago that several friends said was wonderful, but from my observation, what it did was make them stagger around the room and fall down, usually clearing a table of drinks in the process, just before throwing up.

In 2005, there were five factories in China licensed to manufacture and export Ketamine, an unknown number operating illegally in other countries, and according to the U.S. Drug Enforcement Agency, active throughout the region, seizures where illegal had increased by over five hundred percent in the past few years. *Time* magazine reported the same year that it had overtaken Ecstasy in Hong Kong clubs and said that of all users under the age of twenty-one, fifty-nine per cent were using K, mostly in pill or capsule form.

Finally, Viagra and Cialis and all the copycats from India and China often were taken as "aphrodisiacs" by men who didn't really need them, but used them to make a good thing even better. So, too, cocaine, the well-known byproduct of the South American coca plant, its proponents citing the added benefit of increasing erectile longevity through its application to the head of the penis, dulling sensation (and premature ejaculation) in much the same way its chemical cousins Novacaine and Procaine were used as local anesthetics in dentistry.

Last but not least were "poppers," the street name given a family of compounds named alkl nitrites, the original, amyl nitrite, being used for many years to combat spasms of the heart called angina, a prescription medicine that came at that time in small ampoules that you "popped" to release vapors that were then inhaled. In time, cardiac patients were given nitroglycerin tablets instead and the non-prescription sale of nitrites was made illegal. The chemistry was fiddled with and butyl nitrates were the result, sold in small brown, screw-top bottles as a "room freshener" or "video head cleaner" and appropriately called things like Rush or Jolt.

Poppers were not without risk. They were branded dangerous for heart patients and the liquid was as flammable as the high octane fuel it smelled like. Repeated use burned the membranes of the nose. Headaches were common, as well. And in 2005, they were illegal everywhere in Asia except Taiwan.

As a sex enhancer, the effect was to cause all of the muscles of the body to relax (making anal intercourse easier), but most importantly, to bring on vasodilation, or relaxation of the blood vessels, sending oxygen-rich blood to the brain, releasing inhibition, increasing lust, encouraging a sense of raw animal sexuality. The hit lasted only a minute or so, but if you had an orgasm during that moment in time, you were a fan for life.

Chapter twenty
Gooey Is Good

If I thought the potions in ancient Asia were amazing—demonstrating to what lengths a man, and to a lesser degree a woman, would go to enhance sex—I hadn't gotten to the lotions yet. And again it was in India where the various medicines "for external use only" exceeded those found elsewhere, both in imagination and credibility.

One from the *Kama Sutra* (where else?) called for "a mixture of the leaf of the plant *vatodbhranta*, of the flowers thrown on a human corpse when carried out to be burnt, and the powder of the bones of a peacock." While another was "made of leeches, but only of such as live in water. You put as many of them into a bottle as can be got in, and fill it up with oil. Then expose the bottle to the sun, until the heat of the same has effected a complete mixture. With the fluid thus obtained the member is to be rubbed several consecutive days, and it will, by being thus treated, become of a good size and of full dimensions.

"Another way is to crush leeches with oil, and rub the

member with this ointment; or, if it is preferred, the leeches may be put into a bottle, and, thus enclosed, buried in a warm dunghill until they are dissolved into a coherent mass and form a sort of liniment, which is used for repeatedly applying to the member. The member is certain to greatly benefit by this."

The recipes went on and on. "By rubbing the phallus on all sides with bristles of (Kandalika) insects born on a tree (and caught by a pair of tongs), and massaging it thereafter with oil for ten nights, a man can enlarge his phallus. He should repeat this process until it becomes swollen to the required size, and then he should lie on a cot and cause it to hang down, through a hole in the cot. He should then anoint it with cool concoctions to allay the pain (otherwise the pain and swelling will continue)."

There was a recipe for increased sexual vigor—this was one of my favorites—that suggested I melt down the fat from the hump of a camel for use as a lubricant, another that urged me to rub "the virile member and the vulva with gall from the jackal."

There were unguents recommended for the lady's pleasure, too.

One said the man with "a small member, who wants to make it grand or fortify it for the coitus, must rub it before copulation with tepid water, until it gets red and extended by the flood flowing into it, in consequence of the heat; he must then apply a mixture of honey and ginger, rubbing it in carefully. Then let him join the woman; he will give for her such pleasure that she objects to him getting off her again.

"Smearing the vagina of a woman belonging to the Cow-elephant type [meaning she had a large vagina] with the juice of the (white) Kokilaksha fruits results in the contraction of the organ within one night. On the other hand, the vagina of the Deer-type of woman [a small vagina] can be made to expand within one night if it is treated with the paste made from powdered Padma (white), Utpala (blue), Sarjaku, Sugandha, and honey."

The good news is that I had no idea what most of these ingredients were and I was back home in Thailand by the time I got to that part of the various *Kama Sutra* translations; and I figured those herbs or roots or whatever they were, were in India and for all I cared, there they and the leeches could stay.

The bad news is that there were plenty of other pastes, ointments, and unguents with ingredients that not only were identifiable but also readily available, some no more distant from my penis than my pantry. I just hoped that in combination none of them would require me to dangle my willy through a hole in a cot and bathe it with something cold to halt the pain.

The *Kama Sutra* was not my only source of sex-enhancing recipes. The lesser-known but also esteemed *Ananga-Ranga*, or *Hindu Art of Love*, also dealt with courtship, marriage, coital technique, and the proportions of the genital parts—some thirty-three different subjects in all, for which one hundred and thirty recipes and prescriptions were spelled out.

The Chinese classics were no less helpful. Tung Hsuan Tzu wrote in *The Art of the Bedchamber*, published during the Ming dynasty: "Obtain three fen [0.36 grams] of top quality *jou ch'ung jung* [a Chinese herb] and two fen of top quality *hai tsoa* [a kind of seaweed] and grind them into a powder. Find a white dog born in the First Moon of any year. Use the secretion of its liver to mix the powder into a form of paste. Apply the paste to your jade stem three times. At dawn the following day draw some fresh water from the well and wash it off. Your jade stem will definitely grow three inches longer."

If so many of the ingredients were unknown to me as to make experimentation unlikely, I still had that little bottle of skink oil that I'd purchased in Bangkok, the vendor suggesting a daily painting of my penis for ten days to do I wasn't sure what. I'd also picked up a small bottle of turtle oil in Jakarta while investigating the *jamu* scene there that promised on the label "To Stiffen Vital Organ Muscles, Make It Bigger and Harder Than Before." (I was further advised to massage it into the "vital organ" for about fifteen minutes every morning before taking a bath.) I further had a bottle of Crocodile Massage Oil I'd picked up at the Crocodile Farm outside Bangkok.

I decided before I took those three lotions for a test drive, I'd review some of the simpler external applications. The lubricants designed to ease the friction that is so much a part of intercourse hardly needed much exploration and their universal availability hardly made them seem particularly Asian. They included the saliva and genital juices provided by nature, or commercial substances that included petroleum jelly (such as Vaseline), a lighter petroleum distillate (baby oil), or some form of vegetable oil (olive and soy oil, the only two approved for use by my cardiologist, although anything else slippery will do).

What we're talking about here is anything that can be applied externally for increased sexual pleasure. While researching this book, it occurred to me that I had a variety of sauces on my kitchen shelves and in my fridge, just as I was sure that millions of other Asians did. Did they ever experiment?

And what about Tiger Balm, the salve made in Singapore from Menthol, Camphor, Cajuput, and Olive Oil (with a bit of clove and mint) used for the relief of muscular aches and pains, strains, and insect bites? Nicholas Bornoff in his book *Pink Samarai* said it was used on the clitoris in Japan.

And what if I made a poultice using the numerous fragrant and zesty herbs and fruits so bountifully displayed at my neighborhood market? The penis has been compared to a banana; what if it actually *tasted* like one? In Singapore I bought durian-flavored condoms. Wouldn't ointments for the men and douches for the ladies—and body rubs for both sexes—made from other Asian fruits and herbs offer something as well, using fresh mango, guava, or ginger, Chinese parsley (coriander) or cardamom?

This chapter was turning out to be fun, after all. When this notion came to me, my wife was shopping and I called her on her cell phone.

"Hey, love," I said, "pick up some basil, okay, and maybe some pineapple and dragon fruit."

It was time to try the skink, turtle, and crocodile oil.

The skink, I learned, was one of the most common lizard types and since the oil was purchased in Bangkok, I figured it was the Speckled Forest Skink, whose range stretched from Pakistan and India through Thailand and Indochina and down to the northern Malaysian peninsula. Further research revealed the skink's culinary use in parts of the Middle East and Africa (where it was filleted, soaked in beaten eggs, seasoned, and fried in olive oil), and in ancient Rome where its snout and genitals were pounded together, mixed with herbs and served in wine. While the show-off Persians mixed the skin with amber, ground pearls, saffron and opium. It was also mentioned in *Arabian Nights* as a "seed thickener." Yes, that seed.

Turtles, like skinks and so many other reptiles, have ancestors that date back to the dinosaurs and maybe that's part of the appeal, the longevity, the strength to keep going, no matter what. *The Oxford Companion to Food* said in describing the eggs of one species of turtle that they "may be as large as tennis balls and have a reputation—shared with the smaller eggs of many other species—as an aphrodisiac." I encountered capsules containing turtle in both powder and oil being hawked at one of the upscale malls in Pattaya, large signs advertising the medicine's ability to treat "deficiency sex function and impotence." One to two capsules, twice a day.

The turtle oil I now held in my hand I bought in Indonesia. The liquid was what an "oil" was supposed to be, viscous—thick like any cooking oil, or hair oil for that matter, and somewhat sticky—and I guess it smelled of turtle; imagine musty and swampy in a single whiff. I tried the skink oil later in the day and it offered more of the same: slippery essence of dinosaur. I thought both were excellent lubricants, but that's all, and quite overpriced as such.

The crocodile "oil"—so called on the label—was firm, rather than liquid, about the consistency and color of tan shoe polish. It smelled of camphor or eucalyptus, which turned out to be among the ingredients. As a lubricant I'd give it a Two or Three on a scale of One to Ten, but the cold-hot effect that reminded me of Tiger Balm bumped it up to an Eight.

Chapter twenty-one
The Sweet Smell of Success

I didn't think getting massaged with what are called "essential oils" was going to offer the erotic treat that writers of books about aromatherapy and owners of the new spas across Asia claimed. It sounded like a sweet-smelling scam to me. And an expensive one, at that.

Still, when upmarket spas started popping up across Asia, many of them connected to five-star resorts and offering aromatherapy, I thought I should check it out, at least do a Google search on the subject. The more I got into it, the more sources I checked, human as well as on the Net, the more the practice of using volatile plant oils for sexual benefit sounded like fragrant crap.

Much of the information was damning, both from within and without. Not only did the skeptics demand some sort of scientific backup to the advocates' claims, the therapists failed to provide it, wrapping themselves instead in glowing testimonials by satisfied customers and miraculous anecdotes, none of which could be verified.

That's not all. While some aromatherapy types promised the world, others promised nothing at all. After articulating a strong case for cosmetic, massage, and olfactory aromatherapy, one website shot itself in the foot by saying, "The results of Aromatherapy [capital "A" not mine] are very individual. While there is general agreement about the actions of certain oils, Aromatherapy texts may vary in their descriptions of the properties and characteristics of an essential oil. In addition, no two people are affected by the same essential oil in the exactly the same way. Even the same person can be affected differently by the same oil depending on surroundings, time or day or mood."

No one cited any control studies. Aromatherapists also quoted each other, or sixteenth-century botanists (one of whom said lavender was a panacea for epilepsy, apoplexy, and mental problems). Nor did it help convince skeptics like me when aromatherapy was embraced by the same bunch of New Age people who had tried to give "alternative" health practices like bioharmonics and crystal power a good name. I didn't buy any of that, either. My Khmer-Thai wife's belief that she could pick a winning lottery number that came to her in a dream seemed more plausible.

Three book titles—*Scents and Nonsense: Does Aromatherapy Stink?* (1997) by **Cheryl A. Sweet**, *Aromatherapy: Making Dollars Out of Scents* (2000) by **Stephen Barrett, M.D.**, and *The Business of Aromatherapy: The Insider's Guide to Success* (1999) by **Katherine Graf Jenkins**—seemed to say it all for me. Sweet quoted aromatherapists as saying essential oils were the "soul or spirit of plants," that essential oils had a "spiritual dimension" that could restore "balance" and "harmony," as well as improve sex. While Barrett, after commenting on the "dubious claims...dubious 'certification'...and insufficient regula-

tion" of the new industry, said "pleasant odors can be enjoy-
able and may enhance people's effort to relax. However,
there is no evidence that aromatherapy products provide
the health benefits claimed by their proponents." Ms.
Jenkens, on the other hand, suggested it was a better way to
wealth (for women; the audience here is female) than, say,
selling real estate. But only if they became aromatherapists
and opened a spa.

Much of the criticism was keyed to "confused causation."
What this meant was that when an aromatherapist claimed
that if you relax for several minutes in warm bath water to
which had been added a few drops of essential oil, you
would emerge from the tub feeling better than you did
before getting into it. But what caused the happy mood? The
warmth and floating sensation contributed by the water, the
time spent supine and naked, a few drops of some scented
oil, or some combination?

While it was true that in France aromatherapy was incor-
porated into mainstream medicine and some essential oils
were regulated as prescription drugs, and in several other
countries they were included in the national pharmacopoeia, most of the rest of the world smiled tolerantly when
the subject came up. Like so many other alternative therapies, spreading around the globe like a yeast, aromatherapy
had not been subjected to controlled, double-blind studies—the common explanation being that there was little
incentive for pharmaceutical companies to do so if the
results of the studies were not patentable. In other words,
why spend a small fortune testing something that everyone
else can then duplicate if it had any medicinal worth?

All the product attached to the word further made me
more suspicious. Along with all the new spas came schools,
some offering courses that lasted a hundred and fifty hours!

With a nicely framed certificate awarded at graduation. Holistic health centers devoted space to the display of diffusers, lamps, pottery, candles, pendants, earrings (earrings?), shampoos, skin creams, lotions, bath salts, shower gels, et cetera.

Still, I didn't close the door. Living in Bangkok, I was exposed to bad smells often and recognized how easily a good one could change my mood. Asia had many pleasing scents and I cherished them when I encountered them. The incense burning in Buddhist temples (and in my home), the crushed cloves in Indonesia's *kretek* cigarettes, the nightblooming jasmine, the coriander (Chinese parsley) and basil and lemongrass in the Southeast Asian cuisine, these and many more were part of what made the Orient exotic, sensual.

I also had to acknowledge the role played by essential oils and oleoresins in the food industry. At a food show in Bangkok not long ago, I collected information from a company in Kerala, India, Synthite Industrial Chemicals Limited, that offered essential oils made from black pepper, cardamom, celery, clove, cumin, cinnamon leaf, coriander, curry leaf, dill, fennel, garlic, ginger, mace, asafoetida, mustard, nutmeg, sandalwood, green and white pepper. Along with oleoresins for many of the same herbs and spices, as well as cocoa, rosemary, turmeric, vanilla, and onion. All probably worked in the food industry.

But would specific *aromas* (rather than flavors) have real effect? Surely, it was a good idea to *inhale* medicine; didn't asthma inhalers work? Oxygen entered the bloodstream, after all, so why not send some medicinal scents along with it? It was also accepted that the skin was a good transmitter, so the aromatic baths, creams and ointments, and massage seemed a good idea. Would—could—this turn me on?

I knew that I had to take aromatherapy for a test ride. After all, my own publisher for a while had a book in the shops called *Aromatherapy for Lovers: Essential Recipes*.* If not to myself, I owed it to him to take off my clothes and let someone massage me with the highly concentrated liquids extracted from some of the flowers, leaves, resins, barks, roots, seeds, twigs, berries, rinds, and rhizomes of some of Asia's more fragrant plants. How awful could that be?

But first, I did some more research, learning that, according to Sarah Porter and Joanne Rippin, authors of the beautifully photographed *Aromatherapy Massage* (2002), the use of aromatic herbs and plants in medicine went back six thousand years to China, and found a real home a thousand years later in Egypt when priests mixed magical potions and "essential oils gradually permeated all levels of society." Ayurvedic medicine also prescribed numerous aromatics and in the twelfth century with the return to Europe of the first Crusaders, perfumery was reintroduced to Europe and, they claimed, "records show that aromatics were used as protection against the plague and the low incidence of death among perfumers suggest they were to some degree effective." The Black Death killed half of Europe's entire population. Were Porter and Rippon saying a nice smell prevented it from killing more? At this point, I was ready to hang it up.

I stayed the course and further learned that the modern father of aromatherapy was a French doctor named René-Maurice Gattefossé. After a laboratory accident in 1928, he conveniently plunged his badly burned hand into a vat of lavender oil, and when he noticed how well it healed, thus began the modern age of aromatherapy. Today in France,

---

* A book that had gone out of print by the time I started this one; not even my publisher had a copy, so I am unable to quote from it.

medical students are taught how to prescribe essential oils and in the U.K., hospital nurses use aromatherapy to treat patients suffering from anxiety and depression and to make terminal care patients more comfortable.

What, you may reasonably ask, has this to do with sex? Everything, according to aromatherapy supporters. Porter and Rippen suggested a blend of the oils of black pepper, cedar wood, clary sage, fennel, frankincense, ginger, jasmine, rose, and sandalwood. They, and everyone else, also heartily recommended *ylang ylang (Cananga odorata),* an oil derived from the flowers of a tree native to Madagascar and the Philippines and now cultivated in Sumatra and Java. In Indonesia, the blossoms are scattered on the beds of newly married couples. (A trick I tried in my romantic youth, when I sprinkled rose petals over the sheets of my girlfriend. I don't recall if it enhanced what followed; what I do remember is that it stained the bedding permanently. Sorry, Judy.)

Essential oils usually are produced by distillation and are either inhaled or absorbed during a massage once the oils were dissolved in alcohol, emulsifiers, or, most commonly, fats. This allowed them to penetrate the skin easily and enter the body by mixing with the fatty tissue. During the massage, a few drops of one or more oils could also be added to a bowl of hot water, adding fragrance to the room.

It was time to meet the essence and "soul" of Asian botany.

There were too many spas in Thailand to count and the one I selected was in a five-star hotel in Bangkok—never mind which one, I visited nearly a dozen and they all looked pretty much alike. Attendants dressed in white. (Faux medical.) Sprays of cut flowers in the reception, a promise of good scents to come. Bottles of colorful liquids on display. And once inside one of the luxurious rooms, a tub big enough to move into, with fake gold fixtures and towels so fluffy they looked like they'd been made from whole rabbits.

I did not identify myself as a writer and because I paid for the experience, I figured I could say what I wanted to say, regardless of how I felt on exiting. All I specified was that the treatment include the use of *ylang ylang (Cananga odorata)*, the blossoms of an evergreen tree that seemed to be aromatherapy's No. 1 aphrodisiac.

We talked for a bit first. The therapist, a lovely young Thai woman with quirky but understandable English, told me that the essential oil came from the yellow flowers of a tree native to Madagascar and the Philippines and cultivated now in Indonesia. She said I might notice accelerated breathing and palpitations, but not to worry, it was a prelude to a feeling of peace and sensuality. Would I like to have the oil added to my bath water, she asked, or would I like a massage. I told her yes.

I removed my clothes and sank into a voluptuous tub and following a lovely soak, I moved to a table and had my body massaged.

"What thinking you?" the young woman asked from outside the massage area as I dressed. She knew damned well what I thought, and to drive that message home, as I paid the outrageous sum requested, I said, "Could I come again next week?"

Scents of Seduction

There was a time when I was I was led around by my nose even more than I am now. I was a sucker for perfumes and I can still recall the scent worn by my eighth grade girlfriend, Beverly; if I encountered someone wearing that perfume today, I'd probably experience a flashback and ask her how she was doing in Miss Turnly's English class, and then try to convince her we should do something up close and personal, right there in the elevator.

That, of course, is what perfumes and colognes are supposed to do: give the human body a pleasing scent that engages a potential partner's attention, that may lead them sooner or later to bed. It is no coincidence that some of the best known and most successful perfumes over the years have been called Joy, *Eau sauvage*, Opium*, Poison, Paris, Magie Noire, Dolce Vita, Femme, and Le Male, or that in today's market there are perfumes bearing the names of Jennifer Lopez, Paris Hilton, Beyonce Knowles, Britney Spears, Sarah Jessica Parker, and David Beckham. (David Beckham? Eau de Locker Room?)

When it comes to jargon and so-called "science," the creation of commercial scents outpoints the making of wine. Not only may perfume oils contain tens to hundreds of

---

* Opium, a popular Yves Saint-Laurent perfume introduced in 1977, was banned by the Chinese government in 2000, following consumer complaints that its brand name sent an improper message to youth. A spokesperson for the perfume said its name was "meant to be naughty and suggestive, like Christian Dior's Poison." It should be noticed that at the same time, China began producing for export a counterfeit version of the perfume.

ingredients, they are grouped into seven olfactive "families"—floral (fragrances dominated by the scent of one or more flowers), *chypre* (a scent reminiscent of apricot and custard built on a base of bergamot, jasmine, and oakmoss), *fougere* (emphasizing lavender, *coumarin*, and oakmoss, creating a sharp herbaceous and woody scent), leather (featuring honey, tobacco, wood, and wood tars; remember English Leather and Russian Leather?), woody (think sandalwood and cedar), Orientals or ambers (blending vanilla with animal scents), and citrus (just what the name implies).

Into these complex concoctions go flowers (the largest source of aromatics), leaves and twigs, roots (ginger is a biggie in this category), rhizomes and bulbs, seeds (such as coriander, nutmeg and mace), fruits, woods, bark, resins, and lichens and moss, and from the animal world, liquids extracted from the odorous sacs of the Asian musk deer and civet cat, honeycomb, and, perhaps most renowned, ambergris, described by *wikipedia* as "lumps of oxidized fatty compounds, whose precursors were secreted and expelled by the Sperm Whale"—more commonly known as vomit.

The pungent glandular secretion of the male musk deer, found in Afghanistan, Bhutan, India, Nepal, and Pakistan, probably more than any other scent has been linked to sex due to the presence of androstenol, claimed to be a sex-attractant pheromone; thus, its use in male colognes and after-shaves and potions that are touted in the back pages of skin magazines as infallible female lures. Historically this animal has been in such demand by perfume manufacturers that the species is now on international protection lists and a synthetic musk has been developed. Unfortunately, this has not ended the population decline, as there always seems to be a market for the "real thing."

Most aromatics use a mixture of alcohol and water as a solvent, which upon application disperses, leaving the fragrance to slowly evaporate. Perfumers use the musical analogy of "notes" to describe a perfume's effect, reminding me of all the snooty jargon used in the wine business. When you smell a perfume in a store, you smell the "top note" first, which disappears quickly; these are usually described as "fresh," "assertive," or "sharp." The "heart" or "middle notes" follow, these "mellow" or "rounded" scents lasting between thirty minutes to a couple of hours. Finally come the "base notes" which in some cases can linger for days.

I just remembered the name of the perfume my eighth-grade girlfriend wore. Chantilly. Beverly, if you read this, my email address is at the beginning of the book.

Chapter twenty-two
Ragas for Lovers Only

A young man named Xi crept up on his girlfriend's home in the mountainous village in northern Laos. It was the Hmong new year. Courting season. Earlier in the day he and other young men in the village had taken positions opposite an equal number of young women and tossed a soft, black cloth ball back and forth. It was part of a centuries-old courtship ritual.

The Hmong surely were Asia's best known ethnic minority, the result of their participation in America's fight with Vietnam. When the U.S. decided the hell with it and went home, guilt prompted the country to take some fifty thousand Hmong refugees along. Young Xi had no memory of this in 2004 as he approached his girlfriend's home. He hadn't even been born when the war ended and he, like uncounted thousands more, were still in the remote Laos hills.

Squatting quietly in the dark outside the part of the house where he knew his girlfriend slept, Xi whispered to her through the spaces between the rough planks of the wall and played simple melodies on a small jaw harp fashioned from bamboo, another ancient tradition. She then exited the house—her family fully aware of what was happening, but showing no condemnation or interference—and went with the young man into the nearby woods. There, they spread a courting blanket, a prized possession for all eligible bachelors, and consummated their relationship.

When I was growing up in the U.S., passing through the hormone storm that goes with adolescence everywhere, a popular long-play album of the time was *Music for Lovers Only*. Although the producer, Jackie Gleason, a comedian best known for his weekly show *The Honeymooners*, could neither read nor write music, he had an approach to recording popular songs with moody, string-heavy orchestrations and that LP went on to sell half a million copies, a phenomenal figure for the time. Another twenty albums followed, with titles that made no secret of the music's intent: *Music to Change Her Mind; Opiate D'Amour; Champagne, Candlelight & Kisses*; and *Aphrodisia*.

This was music that we—my fellow innocents and I—were led to believe would put the young ladies who were the objects of our fantasies (and lust) "in the mood." Just as young Xi's twanging jaw harp would do in Laos years later.

It didn't work for me. Maybe there were too many violins. And not enough rhythm. And maybe we weren't so innocent, or soon would not be. Because precisely as the fat comedian whose catchphrase was "A-waaaaaay we go!" was killing us softly with violins, Elvis and Jerry Lee and Little Richard and their nasty, get-down peers were showing us how music and sex really worked together. "Love and marriage" and "rings and things and buttons and bows" suddenly were replaced by "Work With Me Annie" and "Sixty-Minute Man" and

"Baby, Let Me Bang Your Box" (the box being revealed as a piano in the final verse).

This did not go unnoticed in Asia, where rock and roll didn't exterminate traditional music entirely, but surely put it on the back burner for many and, in time, it came to dominate the popular music scene, as it and its numerous mutant forms still do today. But that doesn't mean traditional forms are lost. However much can be said about the relationship between rock and roll and sex, in Asia as well as anywhere else, some of the traditional music continues to have ardent fans. When Mick Jagger was interviewed in *Rolling Stone* in November 2004 just ahead of the release of a new album recorded live during his band's recent tour, he was asked if there was "anything better than soul music to make love to." He laughed and said, "Well, Indian ragas can be quite good. They're all long…and they all have climaxes."

The Beatles weren't the first to bring Indian music to the West, but they were the most effective. I was working for *Rolling Stone* in the late 1960s when George Harrison held a press conference in Los Angeles to introduce Ravi Shankar and the sound of the sitar, later in the week to be showcased at the Hollywood Bowl and already part of the recorded Beatles sound. Someone asked George what it was about the sitar, and Indian ragas, that attracted him.

"Listen to it," he said in the lilt so identified with Liverpool, "—it makes you feel goooood."

That was what music was all about. It made you feel good. Sometimes it made you cry, as well, but it always—if it was good music—touched you emotionally. Plucked the strings of your heart, as someone said, and grabbed you by the balls. It was one leg in the tripod "Wine, women and song." It made you want to dance and it made you want to fuck.

Music was, in many ways, the ultimate aphrodisiac, in

Asia as it was anywhere else.

It didn't start in India with Ravi Shankar. The *Kama Sutra* gave a list of the arts and sciences a courtesan should have at her command and they included music, dancing, acting, and singing. Right up to the early nineteenth century, wrote Fernando Henriques, a lecturer in social anthropology at Leeds University, in his two-volume *Stews and Strumpets: A Survey of Prostitution* (1961), "The duties of a temple harlot can be regarded as threefold. She serves in the temple, she prostitutes herself either to the priests or to all individuals, and she acts as a dancer and entertainer not only for the temple but for the public."

Henriques said the girls were trained from the age of five. "There were several different kinds of dancing, but the actual art of dancing consisted of six distinct types of movements—the movement of the eyes, movement and action of the features, movement and action of the breast and chest, movement and position of the hands, movement and action of the feet, and acrobatics." They sang and danced twice a day in the temple, the singing "almost always confined to obscene verses describing some licentious episode in the history of their gods." Lest such wonderful creatures seem an aberration, Henriques said that by the 1920s, there were two hundred thousand such temple acolytes, called *Devadasis*, in Madras alone, when the population was just five million.

Others told the same story. "Since virtually the whole realm of cultural achievement was theirs, the bevy of beautiful professional women gave to a royal court an important part of its splendor," Philip Rawson wrote in *Oriental Erotic Art* (1981). "They were leading musicians and performers in the theater for which Sanskrit and Prakrit and Tamil poets wrote so many hundreds of sophisticated plays and dance-dramas.

"Not only did the Devadasis perform in the dance pavil-
ion at temple services for the deity, making music, singing
lascivious songs and dancing lascivious dances to stimulate
his potency, they also did the same in the houses of royalty,
nobility, and the rich. In addition, some would have sexual
relations with male visitors to the shrine. And since they
became Devadasis by performing the rite of marriage to the
god, for them to couple with a man was a powerful way of
stimulating the divinity in him. In India, divine presence is
associated with the sense of deep sexual arousal."

In China, the situation was quite different. Here, women
were not dedicated to the temples as gifts to the gods, but
sold to what were called "flower boats" as slaves. These were
the floating brothels found in ports, many of them moored
side-by-side, offering entertainment with the drink and sex.
Again, dance and music instruction began early, so that the
girls were ready to earn their keep at about age fourteen. The
Chinese brothel performed a function, Henriques said, that
was "unique in the history of prostitution."

"This function aided the development of a special kind of
singing or sing-song girl who entertained in public or in the
privacy of her home. The latter tended to be used much in
the same way as the brothel—as a rendezvous for businessmen. These girls were not, strictly speaking, prostitutes.
Their ambition in life was, as it was for the girls in the flower
boats, to become the concubine of a wealthy man."

How similar this sounds to the karaoke parlors frequent-
ed by businessmen in Japan and Korea and Taiwan and
Beijing today, and in the go-go dance bars in Thailand.

It is the Asian music to which one listens during the actual act of making love that seems most important—calling for
journeys to India and Indonesia for what I think are the most
compelling forms. I can't think of anything less conducive to

use as a background for sex than most of what's called music in Asia today, even when the songs themselves are about sex. The choreographed, sari-garbed whirling dervishes in the Bollywood extravaganzas and the callisthenic-like steps of hip-hop popular throughout Asia make me itchy, but not in the way I wish.

For me, as for Mick Jagger, it's the longer, more insistent, and rhythmical forms that command attention—the sinuous ragas of India and the syncopated gamelan of Indonesia. The forms from India, Java, and Bali may be used to accompany the sexual act, from foreplay to finish.

The word raga—Jagger's favorite Asian soul music—comes from the Sanskrit and means to color with emotion. This is India's "classical" music, thus many of the "songs" have some history attached, although contemporary compositions abound. Broadly speaking, the raga can be regarded as a tonal framework for composition and improvisation that, for western ears, can be somewhat unsettling because of its "strangeness," in much the same way Asia's tonal languages bewilder the same foreign ears. In somewhat the same way that Indian cuisine is divided by geography—northern and southern—so, too, its music, falling into (northern) Hindustani and (southern) Carnatic traditions. Brian Jones and George Harrison introduced the whine, drone, and precise fingerwork of the sitar to the Rolling Stones and the Beatles to great effect and largely through the latter's efforts, Ravi Shankar became an international star, but mainly in a concert hall setting.

People who don't like the traditional orchestral music of Indonesia called gamelan—foreigners again—think of it as sounding like a hundred waiters dropping a hundred trays of silverware down a tile stairwell, one after another, somewhat rhythmically, but mostly painfully. Charlie Chaplin, who visited Bali in the 1930s, wrote in his autobiography that he found the music "cold, ruthless, and slightly disturbing; even the deep, soulful passages had the sinister yearning of a hungry Minotaur." It should be recalled that Chaplin, however noted he was for his activities in the bedroom, was a star of silent films.

People who do like the music indigenous to the islands of Java and Bali prefer the description offered by the Canadian-American composer Colin McPhee, who called it a "shining rain of silver [that] rose at one moment to a fury and fell the next to an inaudible throb." For McPhee, who lived on Bali at the time of Chaplin's visit, gamelan was a joyous part of nature's force, as essential to the islands as the tropical rains that sprayed and drenched the fertile land. Say the names of the principal instruments aloud—*gong, kempur, kempli, kemonog, reyong, trompong, gangsa, chalung, jegogan, kendang* and *chen-cheng*—and you cannot be surprised by what their coming together sounds like. Since nearly all of the kettle drums, bells, gongs, cymbals and xylophone-like instruments are made of bronze, and the hammers are of hardwood, the resulting sound may naturally be loud.

Andrew Toth, the American consular agent in Bali, wrote his doctoral thesis on Balinese music at UCLA and is now so adept as a musician he teaches Indonesians in a school in Denpasar, Bali's capital. "This is the most complex percussion music in the world. When it comes to interlocking parts, abrupt accelerations, sudden stops, displaced accents, highly developed counterpoint and multilayered, polyphonic, synchronized instrumental parts, nobody can touch the Balinese," he says, lapsing into fluent musicology. "Jazz musicians go nuts because they can't count it, and children delight in its rhythmic simplicity."

It's also perfect for lovers. As with ragas, the pieces usually start slow and they build to wonderful climaxes, with numerous starts and stops and changes in between. Just like you know what.

There is one thing more about gamelan that should be mentioned and that is the "battle of the gamelan bands." There are an estimated ten thousand gamelan orchestras on Bali alone and one of the highlights of any year's busy calendar of temple fairs and other local, cultural festivities occurs when two of the musical congregations come together in competition.

Gamelan is a memorized musical form, without improvisation, with every song played note for note and bong for bong the same way every time, no matter which groups perform it. However, the instruments in the competing orchestras frequently are tuned differently by virtue of the fact that they may be crafted by different instrument makers. So when two of the bands meet in competition and are told to play the same piece at the same time in the same place—hundreds of villagers cheering on their favorites like football fans during the European Cup—the musicians who lose their place lose.

And that sounds like a lot of bedroom experiences, too.

Chapter twenty-three
Different Strokes for Different Folks

I came to massage in pain and then discovered the joy.

Back in the 1980s when I was living in Honolulu, a driver ran a red light and smacked me in a crosswalk, breaking a number of bones, including the first lumbar in my lower back. My bone healed and I resumed my everyday life, but as the pain in my lower back continued, I sought help. In the next six months or so, I explored a variety of healing disciplines.

A back surgeon wanted to do exploratory surgery. Another specialist prescribed traction and gave me some complex equipment that left me hanging by my chin from my bedroom door. A chiropractor showed me a film that made it clear that if I didn't start seeing him on a regular basis, I'd probably die. Someone practicing homeopathy said my pain would go away if I'd just take my wallet out of my hip pocket when I drove my car and sat on a piece of board that I was expected to carry around with me. Someone else suggested a regimen of painkillers. On and on.

Finally I called a friend in Los Angeles who was an

acupuncturist and he told me to find a good shiatsu therapist, see her (he suggested a woman) two times a week until
the pain went away, and then see her or another therapist
once weekly for the rest of my life. Not only to get rid of the
pain but to keep my body toned and fit.

Shiatsu is a system of deep tissue, full body massage popularized in Japan in the twentieth century, but most believe
it originated in ancient China, deriving from Zhi Ya massage,
which also is based on acupressure. It's now found just about
everywhere; once, when I was in London, I called the Japanese embassy and asked who they suggested for visiting
Japanese businessmen and the next day a fireplug of a
woman who spoke no English was mauling me with her
powerful thumbs on the floor of the office I was using.

Bottom line: it worked, and for several years I continued
making weekly appointments to have someone massage all
the pressure points, leaving me feeling at the end of the hour
as if I'd been filleted. I told friends it was like taking my car in
regularly for tune-up. It kept me free of pain and my muscles
loose, and by reducing stiffness in one part of the anatomy I
like to think it helped condition me for rigidity elsewhere.
One of the primary benefits of almost any kind of massage,
after all, was improved blood circulation.

When I moved to Asia in 1993, I discovered traditional
Thai massage, a system that combined characteristics of
ordinary massage (stroking and kneading the muscles) with
some chiropractic moves (manipulating skeletal parts) and
acupressure (applying deep, consistent pressure to specific
nerves). The "tune-ups" continued.

I confess I also discovered Thailand's "other" kind of massage parlors, sometimes called "Turkish baths." This resembled traditional massage only slightly. There was body contact, plenty of it, but the phrase "full body massage" now had

a new meaning. After entering one of the establishments and selecting a "masseuse" from the many on display behind a large plate of glass (called a "fish bowl"), I was taken to a private room, undressed, and directed to a low tub where I was lathered and scrubbed from head to toe, the young woman using not only her hands but also her pubic bush as a brush. A bed was waiting nearby. In this fashion, the character of an ancient Thai medical practice was besmirched and the word "massage" sadly became identified in Thailand with sex. I soon stopped going to the baths, but continued my weekly traditional "tune-ups." Still, whenever I told a friend I'd just had a massage, I got that look and a wink.

So, too, it was elsewhere in Asia, in virtually every Asian country, and especially in Japan, where in the mid-1980s, as I was discovering the healing power of shiatsu in Hawaii, various women's Christian movements were exerting pressure in Tokyo to close down what were called *Toruko-buro*, or Turkish Baths. (An outraged Turkish diplomat was enlisted to say there was nothing Turkish about *Toruku*.) The massage parlors were not closed, but the Japan Bath Association held a competition to select a new name and, quoting Nicholas Bornoff in *Pink Samarai*, "after much ponderous deliberation by a panel of judges, the word 'Soapland' won the day."

This doesn't mean that traditional massage is dead. Hardly. There now seem to be almost as many different kinds of "legitimate" massage available in Asia as Japan has sushi, as Korea has kim chee, as China has dim sum. One website, *www.thebodyworker.com/types of massage.html*, lists seventy-eight worldwide, from acupressure to zero balancing, and *www.en.wikipedia.com* says there are one hundred and fifty, many of the best known and some of the most obscure with roots in Asia.

Wikipedia further noted that "Due to the necessary physical contact between the practitioner and the client, sexual arousal is not uncommon, although in most forms of massage this is unintentional." However, the description continued, "Massage can also be a part of lovemaking for many couples and often takes place in the context of sex work." This is called, no surprise, "erotic" or "sensual" massage.

Numerous sources make a further connection to sex, claiming massage release endorphins—an abbreviation of "endogenous morphine," morphine produced naturally in the body—usually to reduce stress or pain. This is the stuff that was called the "natural high" that long-distance runners experience and is also linked to other strenuous workouts such as swimming, aerobics, football, and, yes, sexual intercourse. Its champions refer to "recent studies," but scientists debate whether measurable levels are released in humans; most of the current data comes from animal models which may not be relevant.

Still, massage does have an impressive heritage. Stone carvings in China dating to the Shang dynasty (2300 BC) describe methods for treating infants with massage. Later techniques are believed to have emerged from these basic techniques. To the casual observer the numerous types of Oriental massage may seem to have little in common. In Indonesia, fragrant oils are used; elsewhere, oils are not. In Thailand, the customer changes into pajamas, while in shiatsu street clothes are worn and only the shoes, belt, and jewelry are removed. Treatments are delivered on a mat or mattress on the floor, on a table, or in a chair. Japanese, Chinese, and Indian systems have complex underlying theories that are missing in Thailand and Indonesia. In most systems, silence is maintained but in others the patient and therapist may chat openly. And the masseur's or masseuse's hands (and elbows, knees, and feet) are used in quite different ways.

All the many systems have much in common, however. The skin isn't just a protective wrapping—keeping all those bones and muscles and organs in their proper place—it also is an organ system that regulates body temperature, senses painful and pleasant stimuli, and frequently is the source of sexual arousal, resulting from a partner's gentle touch, a massage, or as a receptor for something applied to the surface. When I consulted *The Merck Manual of Medical Information* (1997), I learned, to my surprise, that rubbing something onto the skin was almost as effective in getting something into the bloodstream as eating or drinking it.

In addition, all types of massage are aimed at restoring balance and harmony and if their stated benefits infrequently mention sexual arousal or preparedness for sex to follow, they are praised for the resultant relief of psychological stress and improved circulation, which can only help make lovemaking more successful. For good sex, in other words, the body should be well-tuned.

Tui Na (which means "push and grasp") is practiced in thousands of departments of traditional medicine throughout China. It is a comprehensive healing system for babies and Olympic champions and—quoting "The Healing Benefits of Oriental Massage" (1999) by Maria Mercati—those "seeking an occasional massage for deep relaxation and the feeling of being pampered, should not choose Tui Na; it is far too vigorous..." As an aid to sports performance and for treating sports injuries, she says it is without equal, but she adds that it "leaves the recipient with a feeling of lightness and of being energized...feeling happier and more at one with him/herself and the world around."

Shiatsu translates into the word *shi* (finger) and *atsu* (pressure) and refers generally to a Japanese pressure therapy used to relieve pain, tension, and fatigue, as well as treat a number of specific problems such as insomnia and digestive upset. Based on traditional Chinese techniques, it acquired its name with the publication of Tenpaku Tami's book *Shiatsu Ho* in 1919 and was officially recognized by the Japanese government in laws passed in the 1950s and 1960s; all shiatsu therapists in Japan must also complete government-regulated instruction. Pressure is applied by the thumbs, fingers, palms, elbows, feet, and knees. In the West, the system has been adapted to follow the principles of anatomy and physiology.

Traditional Thai massage—those seeking it must be sure the word "traditional" is on the shop sign or window—is much inspired by Ayurdevic techniques and it offers something akin to a yoga workout, without the self-discipline, practice, or physical effort that yoga inevitably demands. The feet are washed and the massage begins there, moving upwards, the pace slow and rhythmical as the practitioner applies deep, sustained pressure to soften the muscle's connective tissue skeleton, restoring energy flow. The patient turns over and the massage continues, now from the shoulders to the feet. It ends with some final stretching and a head workout. One hour is nice, two hours and I feel twenty years younger.

Massage plays a key role in Ayurvedic medicine and usually is tailored to the individual's therapeutic needs, as are the oils that are used. In a more general sense, it is believed to relieve fatigue, improve sight, restore skin tone, encourage resistance to disease, and "make one strong," as the Kerala Ayurvedic Health Clinic put it. By increasing the circulation of "vital life fluids, and because of rubbing, pressing, and kneading massage makes the body strong, increases stamina, vitality, and virility." A writer for *The Observer* in London put it another way, describing his visit to an Indian spa in

2003 as "a deeply glamorous, profoundly indulgent way to experience the benefits of the oldest system of medicine in the world."

The system of bodywork in Indonesia that is so closely linked to the herbal remedies called jamu has clear roots both in China and India. Unlike many oil massages, the oil is not there to elicit sensual response or to make the practitioner's job easier; once again, the thumbs push deep into the soft tissue, following the Chinese energy meridians, and the manipulations are centered on the spine, involving some surprising yogic twists. Although Indonesian massage, most commonly available in Java and Bali, appeals mainly to the skin-toning and beauty market (women), I don't think there's a human alive (male or female) who doesn't respond with voluptuous pleasure to the combination of hands, oil, and flesh.

Reflexology, or zone therapy, commonly called foot massage, is a Chinese system that claims the soles of the feet are divided into a number of reflex zones corresponding to all parts of the body. In China, the feet may be soaked in an herbal bath for ten or twenty minutes before the massage begins; elsewhere a cursory wash with soap seems to suffice. The therapist then goes to work with her hands and carved wooden pegs that can hurt like blazes. (Some shops sell reflexology equipment, rollers and the like.) I have never felt any benefit from this form of massage and most scientists and health professionals consider the whole thing a pseudoscience, with no proven link between any part of my foot and my internal organs. I give it this much space in the book only because it seems to be, like aromatherapy, the current Flavor of the Month.

There are many more. Reiki (pronounced "ray-kay") is a Japanese word meaning "universal life energies," although it

originated in ancient Tibet; rediscovered by a Christian sem-
inarian in Kyoto in the 1800s, it is a holistic, hands-on healing system and there is no body manipulation. Jin Shin Do is
another form of acupressure incorporating Japanese meditation techniques and diet. Zhi Ya is similar to Tui Na, but it
focuses more on pinching and pressing at acupressure
points rather than pushing, stretching, and kneading the
muscle tissue. Kobido facial massage is a combination of
techniques derived from Anma, a traditional Japanese massage, designed to improve skin condition, musculature,
blood and lymph circulation, and life-force energy (*ki*).
Tantric massage, developed in Germany, adheres closely to
the teachings of India, where the body is regarded as the
temple of the soul.

In an earlier chapter the use of a Thai herb called *kwao
krua* is marketed as a massage cream that is supposed to
firm and enlarge a woman's breasts. I once had a scalp massage in Denpasar, the grubby little capital of Bali, that lasted
forty-five minutes and came as part of shampooing of my
hair that I rank among the most sensual experiences of my
life; such attention can also be found in Hong Kong. And
throughout Asia, from Tokyo to Taipei and Bangkok to
Beijing, I've seen for sale an array of massage "equipment,"
including not only a vast selection of massage oils (scented,
made from local herbs and fruit, et cetera) but also a number
of simple devices, such as wooden rollers for the back, neck,
and feet; and wasn't South Korea the source of the beaded
seat covers you install in your car so that you can get a massage while you drive?

Chapter twenty-four
The Tao & Tantra of Ejaculation Control

When I was growing up in the West, there was—as there is today—a common "problem" called "premature ejaculation." Generally, female orgasmic response was then and is now slower than the average male's, so this trouble was no less his than hers. If he couldn't stay the course, she'd be disappointed and he might look like a wimp.

It wasn't just a matter of "if it feels good, do it," it was a case of "if it feels good, do it more." More often or longer, it didn't matter—if you wanted to be considered a stud, to yourself or to your pals, you got it up and kept it up and fucked all day or all night. With multiple partners if possible.

I remember that those with "hair triggers" had several boring ways to delay ejaculation. When some guys felt orgasm approaching, they recited baseball statistics. Others counted backwards from one hundred, and still others recited the multiplication tables: "Eight times seven is fifty-six, eight times eight is sixty-four, eight times nine is seventy-two..." And so on.

It may have worked, but I know now—or at least I have a clue—how wrong we were. We had the right idea—duration was the name of the game—but we weren't extending a good time, we were avoiding what we considered its "completion," or, quite literally, its climax. By counting backwards or thinking about how many home runs were hit by any particular baseball player in any particular season, we not only were delaying ejaculation, we were also taking our minds away from what we were doing and we were diminishing—perhaps erasing—most of the good stuff that came from doing it.

It wasn't until the 1990s, when I moved to Asia, that I even heard about Tantra and Tao, physical and spiritual disciplines from ancient India and China that ran contrary to the repressive and hypocritical Victorian, Catholic, and Puritan teachings that seemed to be the cause of too much sexual unhappiness in the West. Where many Christians seemed to say if it feels good, don't do it, or if you do it, do it only for procreation, Tantrists and Taoists espoused the opposite: yes, sex was part of the survival of the species, but it also was to be enjoyed not only for the ecstatic pleasure of intercourse, but also the "oneness" that the man and woman experience through the balance of the *doshas* and of *yin* and *yang*, for the purification of the body that accompanies bliss in physical and spiritual form by cultivating the totality of one's erotic potential.

It sounded good to me, but I had a problem with some of the advice laid out (for Taoists) by our old friend and sexual mentor, the Plain Girl, introduced earlier in the chapter about Traditional Chinese Medicine. She said "each should live according to his own vitality and not try to force the joys of sex. Forcing joy is harmful." This mythical creature wasn't talking here about *delaying* ejaculation, but *denying* it. And how regularly you denied, or retained, it, was determined by the man's age.

Where a robust male of twenty was told he could ejaculate twice daily, she said a thirty-year-old male should cut back to once a day. At forty, the limit was once every three days, at fifty once every five days, at sixty once every ten days, and at seventy years of age, once a month, providing the guy was in good health. In poor health, she said, he should no longer emit semen at all. At age sixty-nine, overweight and a steady drinker who'd had cardiac surgery, this notion did not extend instant appeal to me.

I'd also been raised in the U.S., where Western medicine claimed that men naturally replenished their semen supply after ejaculation and that the male's capacity for producing semen was virtually limitless. It was also commonly believed that the decrease in sexual stamina that came with age was merely the result of growing old, a fact of advancing life that resulted in the faltering of numerous bodily functions, not merely those below the belt.

Who was I to believe?

Dan Reid said in *The Tao of Health, Sex and Longevity* that Tao wasn't just about making sex good, it was about enhancing and prolonging life. "Chinese culture evolved entirely around the fundamental framework of Tao," he wrote, "and today its principles still lie at the heart of all the classical Chinese arts, from philosophy to poetry, calligraphy to cooking, medicine to meditation."

That said, from the consistent and frequent advice offered by Tao teachers, it was clear that "semen retention," or "ejaculation control," formed one of the philosophy's most important pathways leading to that promised good health and long life. The Tang Dynasty teacher Sun Ssu-mo allowed himself only one emission for every hundred copulations, Reid (and numerous others) said, and Dr. Sun lived to the age of 101. The theory was that retaining semen during sexual intercourse increased the "quantity of life-giving, age-retarding hormones secreted in a man's body during sexual excitement," thus allowing the "essential elements of retained semen to be reabsorbed within the man's body", thus "nourishing" all tissues and organs, including the brain.

Taoists said that when frequent ejaculation exceeded the capacity of the body to fully replenish semen, men experienced chronic fatigue, low resistance, irritation and other symptoms of essence and energy deficiency. They also lost all sexual interest in their partners, who may be ready for more. Frequent intercourse with infrequent semen emission, on the other hand, maintained a man's interest in the act as well as his capacity to continue indefinitely, until his partner was fully satisfied.

Good stuff, every bit of it, if it was true. But it didn't stop there. When I asked Dan for comment, outside that which he'd already offered in his book, he said, "Saving semen is only important for men past middle age if they are living some place like Bangkok, where daily ejaculation is almost as common as having a cup of coffee is elsewhere in the world. And it's not a good idea to retain it every time: three-four times a month of letting it out is regarded as a good guideline for most men at that age. The problem with losing semen every day at our age is the fact that the body, regardless of your condition, will always immediately muster its resources to replace semen each and every time it's emitted. A primary source of ingredients for replacing semen is cerebro-spinal fluid, where many of the essential nutrients are stored, so what happens with daily ejaculation past middle age is a progressive weakening and dilution of the cerebro-spinal fluid, which in turn results in memory loss, confusion, and other symptoms of what's commonly known as 'fucking your brains out.' Frequent, especially daily, ejaculation when you are over the age of fifty will definitely lead to brain deficiency (poor memory, slow mental response, depression, et cetera), and also a very weak spinal column. Ejaculation is not in any way a moral, philosophical, or disciplinary issue in the Taoist tradition, it's just a practical allocation of diminishing resources."

I couldn't help remembering all those myths about masturbation. How many adolescent boys in the West were told that if they didn't stop, hair would grow on their palms, or they'd go insane or blind? Hey, I was losing brain cells anyway, along with everyone else. It was a natural and unavoidable part of aging. For me, it seemed a reasonable trade-off for what felt good.

Similar in many ways and no less complex was India's contribution to the subject in the teachings of Tantrism. This is a body of beliefs and practices that existed in Hindu, Buddhist, Jain, Bonpo, and New Age forms, the majority of its practitioners spread across South and Southeast Asia, as well as in China and Mongolia. Since the 1970s, it further gained a reputation in the West that linked the term Tantra with exotic lovemaking practices taught in the Orient. Thus, it developed into a small industry on the Internet that offered workshops and product, including "100 Explicit Position Photos" and "Hours of Streaming Video." It was also embraced by celebrities, Woody Harrelson and Sting among them, in much the same way that Indian gurus attracted the Beatles, the Beach Boys, Mia Farrow, and other stars forty years earlier.

(Some Indian "teachers" welcomed such attention. Remember Bhagwan Shree Rajneesh, the pop guru in the 1980s who became known for his ashram in India where he accumulated a collection of Rolls Royce automobiles, exchanging courses in breathing techniques, yoga, massage, and an atmosphere of free and open sex to young Western travelers in exchange for their trusts funds and bank accounts?)

In its less adulterated Indian forms, Tantra is, like Traditional Chinese Medicine, an all-encompassing system of rituals and remedies aimed at the perfection of the human being. Some believe Shiva was the first Tantric guru. Others merely say that it is at least as old as Hinduism, which started 3,500 years before Christ. And like TCM and its Tao underpinnings, the object of the sex act in Tantra is "oneness" that the man and woman experience during the Ecstasy of prolonged intercourse.

For most men, this requires something not generally regarded as particularly important: ejaculation control. (To return to our theme.) "When a man ejaculates, he is releasing vital essence or energy which is carried out of his body by the ejaculatory fluids," wrote William Collinge in *Subtle Energy Awakening to the Unseen Forces in Our Lives* (1998), echoing the dire advice of Dan Reid. "The temporary feeling of depletion that men have after ejaculation is thus a true representation of what has happened. Men who use Tantric sexual practices that involve semen retention—that is, intercourse without ejaculation—do not experience this depletion of vital essence, and in fact feel more energized afterward. It is like having their batteries recharged or receiving an infusion of vital energy. Plus, they are able to have intercourse more often, for longer periods, and enjoy more potency in the process."

"At bottom," said Philip Rawson in his book *Oriental Erotic Art*, "Tantra accepts that the appearance of the phenomenal universe around each person is generated by the Great Goddess; she is the womb or matrix of inner and outer reality." The first stage toward that person's release was built around worship of the Goddess, first as she takes the form of an icon, in time transferring that worship (called *puja*) to one's creative self. Then barley, fish, wine, and meat are sanctified and eaten, and intercourse takes place between members of the opposite sex, regardless of who is married to whom. "The aim," Rawson said, "is to pass beyond the bounds of convention—but carefully, within a properly sanctified environment."

Dozens of books have been written about Tantra and most have been focused on sex, producing titles that used phrases such as "Yoga of Sex," "The Secret Power of Sex," and "The Cybernetics of Sex and Love." Even Alex Comfort, famed for his bestselling *The Joy of Sex* (1972), wrote a book called *Tantra of Sex*, a subject that he always said was what got him interested in the "art" of fucking in the first place. However scholarly Doc Comfort's works, it's no surprise that such teachings produced not only a shelf full of authors, but also exploitative entrepreneurs and charlatans to appeal to those who thought, wrongly, that Tantra sanctified clusterfucks.

Such people were mistaken. Both Tao and Tantra were otherworldly, concerned with cosmic connections, and the rituals and practices were always presented in a philosophical context, most of them non-sexual. Like most of the herbal remedies suggested for improved health (and sex), they didn't offer quick fixes. Such study was not goal-directed in the sense of seeking orgasm or other immediate pleasures, but rather it adopted a more relaxed, meditative nature, Tao emphasizing the earthly delights that stemmed from the union of opposites, Tantra employing breathing and yoga exercises to move the practitioners in the same direction, both aimed at bringing individuals and partners closer to the spirit of the universe.

That said, for those who didn't wish to sign up for the whole package, the two schools still offered some practical, sort of halfway advice. Dan Reid said the loss of essence and energy due to emission was possible "by learning to 'come lightly' when you choose to ejaculate. Instead of thrusting to a frenzy just prior to ejaculation, approach the brink slowly and gently and savor the exquisite sensation of release, then deliberately 'squeeze off' the urogenital canal with a deep contraction of the anus and penile shaft before the ejaculation is over. This will conserve about twenty-thirty per cent of your semen while still providing the desired ejaculatory release.

"Immediately after emission, rhythmically contract the entire urogenital diaphragm for a minute or two by practicing anal sphincter locks. This tightens up the pelvic floor, which becomes loose and flaccid after ejaculation, and thereby prevents post-coital loss of *chee* [*qi*] through the perineum, anus, and urogenital canal. This exercise is highly beneficial for women as well, because it prevents loss of *chee* through the vagina and encourages sexual energy to move up the spinal channels to the brain."

The alternative, of course, is to say the hell with all that talk about loss of brain cells and recite the multiplication tables while making love.

"Five times four is twenty, five times five is twenty five, five times six is thirty…"

Chapter twenty-five
From Pillow Talk to Pornography

The men in the Bangkok shopping mall matter-of-factly shuffled through the stacks of cellophane envelopes, each showing the photographic artwork of a pornographic video. At this stall and at numerous others, bootlegged copies of the latest video games and software were sold and some of the first-run films from Hollywood were available in the DVD format only days following their theatrical release in America. This also was where those seeking entertainment could find the largest selection of DVDs and VCDs rated XXX.

For the Japanese businessmen working in the city, and others who were so inclined, there were videos from Japan, most of them live action but many what are called *hentai*, animated renditions of the popular cartoon books called *manga*. Young women with impossibly large Western eyes and breasts were depicted with older men with impossibly large penises, the men spouting like volcanoes, their partners often crying and bleeding.

For the Thais there were homegrown discs of every sort,

some of them showing Thai couples, others showing young Thai women with Caucasian foreigners.

For everyone, there was a little of everything—all of it copied on high speed machines from videos made in Europe and the U.S. that were zipped to Thailand by satellite or physically carried in by plane. There were gay and lesbian videos, as well, and always a few involving dogs and horses and other special kinks. The VCDs cost $2.50, DVDs, which tended to be more carefully copied, a dollar more.

The display envelopes were empty and numbered. Customers flipped through the envelopes and told the clerk which numbers they wanted and after handing over the money were told to come back in twenty minutes. The discs were not on the premises, to escape confiscation by the porn police, but ordered by phone and delivered by a runner who came from the source, perhaps no farther away than a van in the building's parking garage.

All forms of pornography were illegal in Thailand, but like any other behavior or illicit mercantile activity in the Land of Smiles, the laws were not strictly enforced. In fact, pornography was banned across much of Asia—forgetting Japan, where it was sold unashamedly in vending machines and men read it openly on commuter trains, and in China and Hong Kong, where the laws forbade its sale to minors—but of course it was always available if you knew where to look and, unlike in the West, it was sold at a bargain price.

As elsewhere, it was purchased in Asia for self-amusement and as an aid to sex with others. As I was writing this chapter, Durex, the world's largest condom manufacturer, announced that Thais topped a global poll in 2005 for using porn during sex, with sixty-seven per cent of Thai men answering an online questionnaire endorsing its use as a stimulant. Elsewhere in Asia, the survey put Taiwan in the

Number Two position with fifty-seven per cent, followed by Malaysia and Hong Kong (tied for third at forty-nine per cent), Indonesia at forty-four per cent, Singapore at forty-three, Vietnam at thirty-eight, India at thirty-seven, Japan at twenty-two, and China at sixteen. (Japan's low placement seems surprising, but maybe Japanese men don't think all that kink is pornographic.) The global average was forty-one per cent.

And of course it was available nearly everywhere in Asia on the Internet, although several countries have been effective in blocking numerous websites.

Once again, the Indians, the Chinese, and the Japanese led Asia when it came to sex, and in this instance it was in the development and marketing (and acceptance) of pornography. There will be those who criticize me for what I'm about to call porn. That's "erotic art," not porn, they'll insist. Well, my dictionary defines pornography as "writings, photographs, et cetera, designed to arouse sexual desire." Art historians agree that the album miniatures commissioned by the Rajput courts in Rajasthan and the Punjab starting in sixteenth-century India and continuing through the nineteenth, the paintings on scrolls and silk in China in the 1600s, and the woodblock illustrations called *shunga* that characterized Tokyo's "floating world" beginning at the same time were created to arouse. And that, for me, means the "art" was also pornography, as well as an aphrodisiac.

In *Oriental Erotic Art*, Philip Rawson wrote, "The styles of Indian erotic art emphasize the eternity, sublimity and vastness of their subject matter. Chinese arts, with their subtle metaphors and allusions, lead the mind into a world woven together by invisible threats of force and significance; while Japanese art, especially that of Edo [seventeenth-century

Tokyo], conveys a sense of the splendor of sex, but reflects at the same time a Buddhist view of the phenomenal and transitory in that splendor."

Rawson got down to cases when he added, "First of all, there is no doubt that they were meant to stimulate sexual response. This is obvious in the case of the picture albums and scrolls of lovemaking techniques intended for the use of young lovers. But all Eastern erotic art is also meant to convey what it feels like to be filled with desire."

Following the trail blazed in the *Kama Sutra* and other early texts, including the *Bhagavad Gita* (revealing Krishna at lascivious play), as well as the stone temple carvings that dated back to the tenth century, the miniature Indian paintings, most smaller than six by nine inches (fifteen by twenty three centimeters) depicted sexual variety and dexterity. Not only were many of the positions described in the *Kama Sutra* given artistic dimension, showing couples and groups engaged in manual and oral play and intercourse, but the subjects in this book and Rawson's slimmer but also heavily illustrated *Erotic Art of India* (1982), also were shown enjoying sex while riding on horses, camels, and elephants, while smoking hookahs and drinking wine, while feeding peacocks and shooting deer.

Some pictured foreign men with Indian women. In one painting a prince was having sex with five women at once, two with his hands, two with his feet, and the fifth more conventionally. In another, the naked lovers were fornicating with what appeared to be the woman's small son pulling at her hand to get her attention, illustrating how, within the privacy of the palace, sex was not thought to be something to hide from children. In one painting, a woman was having sex not on top of a horse but under it, and with the horse!

These unbound "albums"—really, more a stack of paintings—were intended for aristocratic households and often served as instructional manuals. Today, they are in museums and on the walls of wealthy collectors. (Most of the paintings in Rawson's book of Indian art came from the collection of Victor Lowndes, who was Hugh Hefner's partner in *Playboy*'s early years.)

China's answer to the *Kama Sutra* was a collection of scrolls, now a book, called *The Golden Lotus*. As in India, the scrolls were created for the upper classes and used that society's personal style and home settings as background for the acts of sex; making clear the connection to the privileged class, all the women in the illustrations had bound feet. Often, the scrolls were accompanied by detailed instructions. One dating from the fifteenth century said, "The man has two women lie on the bed, in each other's arms, one lying on her back and the other lying on top of her, stomach to stomach, so that their public regions are touching. Then the women have to rub against each other, without his help, until the gates of the golden lotus are wide open like the mouths of fish in water.

"The man kneels between their legs and waits until both women approach their climax. Only then does he separate them slightly, stick his pleasure stalk between their pubic regions so that both of them can feel it, and move forward and backward until they reach their climax. This intercourse reinforces the man's muscles and tendons and contributes to the strengthening of his virility."

This exercise was called "The Intercourse of the Fluttering Fishes." The Chinese gave such flowery names to dozens of positions, again as did the Indians in the *Kama Sutra*. A popular modern version of *The Golden Lotus*, published in Israel in 2002, takes the form of questions being asked of our old friend the Yellow Emperor. His answers often were long and reminded me of the lines from a poem: "How do I love thee? Let me count the ways..." Following the Taoist precepts, his answers often came in list form. There were five passions, ten movements, four forces, eight advantages and seven disadvantages of energy, twelve main points, five signs, eight types of embrace, ten signs of finishing (climax), eight styles of sexual intercourse (or ten, it varied), ten modes of penetration, and thirty sexual positions.

The names of the artists in India and China are not known, but in Edo era Japan—Edo being the name for the city that became Tokyo—many of the painters became stars. Japan was closed to all outside trade (and would remain so until America's Commodore Perry arrived with his warships in 1858); thus isolated, its indigenous art scene and a new-found sexual liberty exploded amongst the growing bourgeoisie. They made cults of Noh and Kabuki theater and engaged in open and promiscuous sex in a neighborhood created for such pleasures, Yoshiwara. (The men did, anyway; the wives, then as now, were expected to stay at home and wipe noses, cook, and clean house, unless as members of the *daimyo*, or privileged class, they could afford servants, and then their role was to manage the servants.)

The most explicit drawings, called *shunga*, or "Spring Pictures," were produced as an inspiration and aid to newly-weds and other inexperienced lovers. Initially the forms were simply drawn and printed in black and white. A second color was added in the eighteenth century, polychrome after that, opening the door to woodblock art that was as beautifully patterned as the voluptuous robes worn by the men and women making love. Sometimes, flecks of real silver and gold were mixed with the paints and the text of the accompanying story was written on the picture itself.

The artwork was quite astonishing, in both the extraordinary attention paid to the genitals and a sense of humor not seen in India or China. Penises were hugely enlarged and veined, vulvas extravagantly pleated—in defiance of Japanese anatomical reality. One picture showed a man with an erection so big, he had to carry it in a wheelbarrow that he pushed before him.

For two hundred years (1660–1860), *shunga* decorated the interiors of the "green-houses" of Yoshiwara, depicting the *geisha* who worked there and many of the popular actors, often in erotic motif. Not all of the art was pornographic; the great Hokusai, deemed one of the most skilled, was known also for his landscapes, including a masterwork titled *Thirty-Six Views of Mount Fuji*. Yet, it is the clinically detailed sex scenes that are remembered and reprinted in slick coffee table books today.

Rawson estimated that at least forty per cent of the total output was "overtly erotic." Much of it depicted the same sexual positions shown elsewhere earlier; the Chinese influence was obvious. But there were rape scenes as well, and male and female homosexual acts, sadism and voyeurism and bondage, and scenes with horses and dogs. Other pictures illustrated relations between women and Buddhist monks and sex between Buddhist nuns. Neither Buddhist nor Confucian morality approved of any of this art, which was the painters' point.

Most important, this was the first erotic art to be reproduced in quantity—thanks to the woodblock technique—and thus it was both widely available and affordable. Many were rented from bookshops. In 1808, there were more than six hundred shops in Edo—approximately one for every 1,500 people—and another three hundred in Osaka. At last, pornography for the masses.

These scrolls and prints from China and Japan were

called "Pillow Books" and it was the *shunga* that influenced what can be seen today. In a little over a hundred years, *Shunga* morphed into *manga*, *anime*, and *hentei*, cartoon forms that soon found multi-million-dollar markets overseas. *Manga* were the comic books, *anime* was the animated cartoon version of those comics, and *hentei* was the pornographic *anime*. In 2004, about forty-five per cent of all books and periodicals sold in Japan were *manga*, and more hundreds of millions of dollars' worth were being exported to or printed in dozens of countries around the world. Not all of it was pornographic—*anime* encompassed many genres, including comedy, action, fantasy and science fiction, and children's stories. But the *manga* and *hentai* that gave Japan its reputation was graphically sexual and, as often as not, violent and degrading to women, especially if they were young schoolgirls.

At the same time, Japan spawned one of world's largest pornographic film industries. In the 1960s, genres called *pinkku eiga* (pink cinema) and *roman poruno* (porno romance) were produced by mainstream filmmakers, including one of Japan's top directors, Nagisma Oshima. One of the oldest film companies, Nikkatsu, released three such features a month for fifteen years, during which time soft porn comprised two-fifths of the country's entire film output. When video production began in the 1980s, the number of adult videos, called AVs, jumped to four thousand a year, made by over seventy companies.

Nicholas Bornoff wrote in *Pink Samarai*, "Most adult videos have the simplicity of the old woodblock print, and an inactive third party, the *shunga*'s perennial voyeur, is also nearly always in evidence. While one of two disport themselves with the star on the mattress, a frustrated third representing the spectator sometimes jiggles around in his underpants, either contorting himself in an agony of anticipation or looking on and languidly masturbating."

It wasn't all so tame. In order to get around the laws banning the depiction of a woman's pubic hair and sexual penetration, the Japanese created *bukkake*, the noun form of the Japanese verb *bukkakeru*, meaning "splash" or "dash." Indeed, *bukkake* is more commonly used in Japan to describe a type of dish, where the toppings are poured onto noodles. In Japanese porn, it depicted a woman—frequently a demure schoolgirl or panty-hosed office lady—being tied up and drenched with semen by dozens of men. Introduced in the early 1990s, it quickly made its way to the West, where the only adaptation was to depict the woman as enjoying it.

As happened in other cities before—San Francisco for its homosexual population, Bangkok for go-go bars and massage parlors, Amsterdam and Hamburg for legal prostitution—Tokyo became known for sex, and this did not always make the country popular elsewhere. By 1999, Interpol estimated that at least eighty per cent of the world's commercially distributed child pornography originated in Japan. *Time* magazine called it "Japan's Shame" and it wasn't until after three years of debate that the Diet, Japan's parliament, made it illegal...although apparently to little effect, as Japanese police found more than three times as many children used as pornographic models in 2005 than a year earlier.

It was also illegal to bring pornography into Japan, but one has to wonder why anyone might wish to.

Chapter twenty-six
The Joy of Mechanical Sex

Adrian Macintosh, a tall, lean, fifty-something expatriate from Scotland living in Taipei, entered the Shanghai Exhibition Center and was completely blown away. In this high-ceilinged space at least half the size of a football pitch, there were hundreds of booths in long aisles taking orders from buyers from around the world (but mainly from Asia, as he soon learned) for dildos, anal toys, vibrators, and other "insertables"; chastity devices; vaginal suckers; nipple enlarger kits with and without pumps; cock rings made from aluminum, neoprene, stainless steel, leather, denim, Velcro, and rubber (in eight colors, some of which glowed in the dark); anal beads; ball stretchers and separating ball weights; cock harnesses; penis pumps (including a double-ended cylinder so two men could pump together); ticklers; herbal aphrodisiacs; lubes and lotions; life-sized inflatable dolls with "realistic" vaginas and penises; plastic vaginas (with and without pubic hair); and for those who wanted to justify with historical precedent that which went into their shopping carts, reproductions of hundred-year-old erotic paintings that served as China's earliest pornography.

Adrian walked the aisles, looking at penis jewelry, videos and printed pornography; there seemed to be no end to it. Most of the signage was in Chinese and Adrian understood not a word of it, his pale face and large frame making him a curiosity; most Westerners who sold sex toys on the Internet did their shopping at bigger trade shows in the U.S. and Germany. But he lived in Asia, so he shopped in Asia. He figured prices were cheaper here, anyway, and when he saw something he thought he'd find a market for on his website, there always seemed to be someone nearby who spoke enough English to make the deal. He then had the product shipped from the Chinese factories to the U.K., where sale and export of such product was legal.

Before he moved to Asia, Adrian sold automobile accessories. He was married then. Now he was not. He had visited Asia many times and decided to set up a base in Taipei. At the time, in 2002, the Internet market was beginning to explode, so when he made his move, he decided to take advantage of it and start selling sex toys in cyberspace. The market wasn't so crowded then.

Some of the booths at the exposition displayed only a few products. Others handed out catalogs with hundreds of items. Adrian looked at fetish wear and lingerie; armbands and gauntlets; bondage restraints; cuffs and collars; spreader bars (that hold your legs apart); metal restraints; straitjackets; bondage hardware and locks; blindfolds; gags and muzzles; hoods and masks (lacing up the back to fit heads large and small); slings and swings; leather clothing; whips, paddles, and crops; pony gear (a most peculiar selection that offered a "pony head bridle set" that made you look like you had your head in a leather feed bag, reins, and a variety of pony-tailed anal plugs); a cocksucker's mirror (that fitted over the penis and balls, laying flat against the tummy so you can watch what you're doing); something described as a "polished aluminum humbler with crusher attachment" and something else that made the expat shake his head: a "parachute ball stretcher with spikes."

Credit cards accepted. Delivery in four to six weeks.

Adrian was amazed. Was this really "Communist China"? It seemed difficult to believe. Maybe all those stories about China opening up to the West were true. If Mao had been put in a grave instead of on display in Tiananmen Square, he'd be spinning in it.

According to *The Guardian* (June 25, 2005), the first "adult health retailer" opened in Beijing in 1993. A dozen years later the capital was estimated to have two thousand such shops, with another two and a half thousand in Shanghai; no neighborhood seemed lacking. "Most of the early establishments were dowdy and staffed by matrons in white laboratory coats, offering potency pills to a largely male clientele," *The Guardian* reported. "But increasing competition is pushing retailers to be more imaginative in their presentation. Public advertising is forbidden, but managers are displaying a more colorful array of products on their shelves and expressing a wider range of ideas about their role.

"But achieving recognition has been a hard slog," *The Guardian* went on. "Before he was able to open Shaki [believed to be the first shop], the owner, Fang Hong, said it took him years to acquire the necessary permits from thirty-six different government agencies. His business, which has since grown at the rate of more than twenty per cent per year, now employs three hundred people during the peak season, before Christmas.

"Casting an expert eye over a range of blow-up dolls, he said Westerners preferred large realistic figures with lipstick and wigs, while his Asian customers tended towards petite inflatables with cartoon faces."

The *Economist* reported (Dec. 24, 2005) that the most successful of China's new sex tycoons was Wu Zhenwang, the owner of an electrical machinery business in Wenzhou, an industrial city south of Shanghai, who changed his career after seeing one of those first shops on holiday with his family in Beijing. He noticed most of the product was imported and high-priced and thought he could mass-produce the stuff for less.

"Thanks to his good connections with local officials (a prerequisite of success for the Chinese entrepreneur) and effective lobbying in Beijing," the *Economist* said, "he was able to get permission to produce them in Wenzhou." He also chose a joint venture partner for what came to be called Wenzhou Lover Health Products, a Japanese sex toy manufacturer, for its experience with relevant technology and contacts in foreign markets.

Wu was China's first manufacturer and even with strong competition today, he and the companies operated by him and his sons control an estimated sixty per cent of the domestic market—some of that represented by their own growing chain of retail shops—as well as a hefty slice of the export market.

The *People's Daily Online*, "Your Gateway to Business in China," reported in 2005 that there were ten thousand Chinese companies involved in the sex product industry, said China was providing seventy per cent of the world's sex toys, and quoted the China Sex Health Committees as saying the annual sales volume of sex products in China in 2003 exceeded $12 billion, a figure that was rising by thirty per cent per year.

This was impressive, but it was nothing really new. It represented a complete turnaround from the days of Chairman Mao's cultural revolution when men and women wore the same boring, blue peasant uniforms and hats and sex was never, ever talked about. But China played an innovative role in the history of sex toys and aids long before Mao and Marx. In fact, China may have been there first.

From Imperial China came the remarkable *ben wa* balls—originally a single ball made from wood, ivory, silver, or jade, and inserted into the vagina to keep a woman's *yin* in a state of arousal, as a prelude to intercourse or amusement when alone. Others unscrewed so that mercury could be poured inside; as the woman walked, the liquid metal moved the ball in a sensual manner. Some contained clappers that made a ringing sound. Still another consisted of two small bags of elastic membrane, joined by a narrow neck, one of them filled with mercury. The empty bag would be inserted into the vagina, the other left outside, and as the woman walked, or pressed her thighs together, the liquid would be forced from the outer bag into the inner one.

During the Han dynasty (206 BC to 220 AD) and again during the Song (960–1127 AD), lesbianism was accepted as a natural result of sheltering a number of wives and concubines under a single roof, thus leading to what Reay Tannahill called in her survey, *Sex in History*, the "harem effect," and the use of dildos.

"All the handbooks warned against too much reliance on these in case they damaged the tissues, a particular hazard, perhaps, with the double kind, a ribbed stick made of wood or ivory," Tannehill wrote. "The 'male' partner inserted one end of the dildo in her own Cinnabar Cleft, harnessed the central portion round her waist by means of silk ties, and used the other end as if it were a Jade Stalk. One medieval novel refers to something called a 'Cantonese groin,' which appears to have been a phallus-shaped sprouting plant that when soaked in hot water swelled and hardened into an excellent dildo."

Still other dildos were crafted from hollow ceramic and filled with hot water to warm the device.

In the Ming dynasty (1368–644 AD), too, a gentleman went onto the "flowery battlefield" with a silk pouch of finely made accessories. In the erotic novel *Golden Lotus*, such implements included "A Silver Passion-clip, A Cap of Eternal Desire, A Sulphur Lust-ring, Medicinal Passion-ribbons, A Jade Dragon-ring, Lust Ointment, and"—giving the armory of love an international flavor—"a Burmese Love-bell," which had nothing to do with Burma.

"Well, what do you think of my battle implements?" our hero asked his lady friend [presenting his Jade Stem in all its glory].

"Struck speechless by the sight, she lay back on the pillows without a reply, fearful yet full of anticipation. Her mouth fell open and her breathing accelerated. Her arms felt weak, but already her knees were rising up from the bed. After attaching the Silver Passion-clip to the Jade Stem, he anointed it well with Lust Ointment, then moved in between her thighs. He tested the position with a brief foray against the Jade Gate, then withdrew and added a Sulphur Lust-ring as well as a yellow and a blue Medicinal Passion-ribbon. His implement thus reinforced, he made resolute entry into the Pleasure Chamber, and she immediately cried out in pain and joy, as if a sword were driving ever deeper into her."

Similarly, in Japan's Edo era, a number of sexual utensils were commonly in use by the period's ruling class. A typical gift from the Higo *daimyo*, a feudal lord in Higo province, to the shogun for his harem was a set of prurient toys that became famously known as the *Higo zuiki*, so named for the dried *zuiki* plant from which the implements were made. Taking the form of a dildo and cock rings of varying design, the fine raffia so meticulously woven as to approximate the most intricate braids of a woman's hair, they were soaked in hot water before use. This caused the fibers to release a juice that was supposed to tickle the vagina into excitement in much the same way as the notorious Spanish Fly. Other descriptions have the gentleman wrapping their cocks with the strands to stimulate and increase its girth.

Many other devices were designed for women who were left alone to amuse themselves. "The Japanese are not moralistic about auto-erotic pleasures," said the anthropologist Ruth Benedict. "No other people ever had such paraphernalia for the purpose." Thus, added Nicholas Bornoff in *Pink Samurai*, "In the Edo period, as evidenced in erotic prints of lonely ladies or nuns, the perennial *harigata* (dildo) reached an apogee. Made of wood or porcelain, the *harigata* was frequently decorated, carved or molded. Sometimes representing Otafuku, folk religion's patron of feminine sexual appetite, or the popular erotic goddess Benten, it was also often sculpted with painstaking anatomical realism, ferociously veined and in sizes with which the real thing could never compete. When made of leather, buffalo horn or occasionally tortoise shell, it could be soaked in warm water prior to use and was reputed to have exactly the right, subtle blend of hardness and flexibility. And whatever it was made of, it also presented the added advantage of never failing to rise to the occasion.

"The common *harigata* was held by hand, but there were other models which could be tied to the heel and which had indubitable merits in a country in which heels are traditionally sat upon," Bornoff wrote. "Moreover, with the *harigata* thus attached, a lady might also loop a cord around her foot and place the other end behind her neck, so that the toy could move around according to the sway of her torso and the ecstatic nodding of her head."

The uncommon *harigata*—perhaps the most uncommon of all—was the classically carved wood Noh mask with a detachable nose.

Many other devices from the same era were designed and used to keep an unwilling willy stiff. Carved from bone, horn, ivory, and wood, some took the shape of sheaths, with windows cut around the circumference to reduce the weight but not the rigidity. Others were simple penis extenders that were fitted onto whatever the man had and tied around the waist. Without inhibition or shame, such implements were openly displayed in homes, on stands identical to those used to hold opium pipes in China and, in Japan, swords and ivory carvings.

Ancient India had its sex gizmos, too. Even the esteemed Vatsyayana in the *Kama Sutra* suggested the use of *apadravyas*, "things which are put on or around the *lingam* to supplement its length or thickness, so as to fit the *yoni*…to be made of gold, silver, copper, iron, ivory, buffalo's horn, various kinds of wood, tin, or lead…soft, cool, provocative of sexual vigor and well fitted to serve the intended purpose."

It wasn't Adrian's first sex product expo in China—that was in Guangzhou a couple of years earlier, when he first started selling this stuff on the Net—but in such a short time the industry had grown up. In 2002, when the divorced Scot moved to Taiwan and started selling sex toys from a website based in the U.K., he didn't have much competition, but today, he said, "you go to the Net and type in the words 'sex toys,' how many sites do you think you get?"

I said I didn't know. Later I did just that on Google and was informed that there were 17.7 million pages waiting for my examination, and in an attempt to narrow the selection, when I typed in "sex toys+China," I got 4.5 million. I also saw a report in the newspaper quoting U.S. researchers as saying ten thousand new websites were registered worldwide every day—two-thirds of them dealing with the sex trade.

"Well," Adrian further asked, "how many pages do you think the average buyer is going to look at before he makes a choice and places an order? Two? Three? Ten? So if you're in the business, you want to be in the Top Ten, aye?"

He paused. "No worries," he then said. "You just pay the man a thousand pounds a day."*

I asked Adrian what his best-selling product was. "The Rabbit," he said, a reference to a vibrator that had a projecting "arm" at the base that stimulated the clitoris when the rest of the device entered the woman's vagina. When it made an appearance on HBO's award-winning show *Sex and the City* as the timid character Charlotte's "new best friend," sales went through the roof. (Singapore didn't permit the series to be broadcast until eight years after its debut and it's still banned in some Asian countries for its candid sexual situations.)

"All of a sudden," said Adrian, "dildos became respectable. You may be surprised to hear this, but fifty per cent of my customers are women and it's because of The Rabbit that comes rolling down the production lines in China."

China may have been the leader, but it wasn't alone. Japan may have been a distant second in Asia's production of

---

* Lest readers be upset by this open bribery, they should know that when they see books on display in bookshops in racks near the cash register, in some of the larger chains the publishers pay very dearly for it.

user-friendly devices when it came to sales, but it was miles ahead in imagination. Here, there was a product called "Pussy in a Cup." Remove the top of what otherwise might pass for a shrink-wrapped cup of dried noodle soup and inside you found, "brimming with a jelly-lotion, this personal massager for men based on the look of a woman's genitals. Insert yourself into the cup and a soft, multi-ribbed sponge will greet you with pleasure. Massage your tension away. May be used as a one-shot or with a condom for multiple use." Only $11.50.

That wasn't all. The same webpage offered a "very soft, large teat you can keep on your desk for whenever you need to squeeze something" ($25); a series of erotic figures of scantily clad women in revealing positions, tied up in bondage poses, measuring 9 cm (3.5 inches) tall ($9 apiece); and a "Girlfriend Knee Pillow" made of soft injected foam, "a perfect replica of a mini-skirted pair of legs to give you comfort when you feel blue" ($108).

At another Japanese website, I found a teddy bear with an outsized penis and, my favorite, a Hello Kitty vibrator.

Condomania

Once upon a time, the condom was sold only in bars and under the counter in businesses catering to men such as pool halls and hair cutting shops, and it was the subject of dirty jokes. Nowadays they have a much better image, one so acceptable that Mechai Viravaidya, known as the "condom king of Thailand" for his colorful and effective efforts to promote population control and AIDS prevention, won the 1994 Ramon Magsaysay Award for Public Service. So strong is his identification with the device that when Thais enter a pharmacy, likely they'll ask for a *mechai*.

One of the things Mechai did was have fun with condoms. He went into Thailand's "red light districts" and onto school campuses with rock bands and had young men and women blow up condoms like balloons and bat them into the audiences. He also opened a chain of restaurants called Cabbages & Condoms that stretched from Bangkok to Beijing; instead of an after dinner mint, customers received a flavored condom. In the twentieth century, the condom was a dirty joke; in the twenty-first it was openly sold everywhere.

From the 1980s onwards, condoms came not only in a rainbow of colors and some that glowed in the dark, they also tasted of strawberry, mint, banana, and durian. They were now ribbed and dotted with bumps and fitted with solid "ticklers" at the closed end to provide more pleasure for women. Some of these ticklers took the shape of cartoon animals. Others were given cute names; China for a time manufactured brands called Clinton and Lewinsky.

Japan topped China with its innovation and packaging. In April 2004 at the International Show of Inventions, Japanese engineers introduced a vibrating condom. A conventional condom was fitted with a ring at the base that contained a battery-operated vibrator, aimed at giving both partners a circular motion along with the usual in-and-out one during intercourse.

The Japanese also produced a series of parody condoms, PokeCon, which except for the slightly altered name looked exactly like Pokemon packaging...the same for the Kit Kat chocolate cookie, renamed KitSack. Other wrappers offered a wide variety of cartoon animals, appealing to Japan's fascination with anything cute.

The biggest challenge of all, perhaps, came in 2005, when the first branded female condom was marketed in Asia. Distributed by the hundreds of thousands in several countries without cost on AIDS Awareness Day, the device looked like a diaphragm with a long skirt and was inserted by the woman prior to intercourse. Manufacturers said it was at least as effective as a conventional (male) condom, but warned that the noises it made in use might take a little getting used to.

"Honey, did you hear something?"

"Yes, what was it?"

"I don't know, it sounded like someone running in mud."

"It sounded like seals barking to me."

Chapter twenty-seven
Surgery: Fact or Phallusy?

I pride myself on the scope of my curiosity, my eager embrace of adventure, my willingness to experiment. When I was researching and writing *Strange Foods* and *Extreme Cuisine*, there was little I refused to put in my mouth. I seldom drew the gastronomical line, confident that, nine times out of ten, I was merely consuming what may have been regarded as weird in the West where I came from, but elsewhere was just called lunch.

I also encountered some things that I wouldn't eat or drink. In researching this book, again I encountered things that were promised to enhance sex that seriously gave me pause. Painting or massaging my willy with an assortment of exotic oils and pastes and submitting it to various stretching exercises and odd devices was one thing, but even the suggestion of anything surgically intrusive made the poor thing get smaller than it already was.

However, this has not been the response of many others who call Asia home and the lengths to which some Asian men are willing to go to increase their size and pleasure are as extraordinary as they are numerous—and, perhaps, as true an indication of courage as they may be of the experimenter's level of quantifiable intelligence.

At the same time, hundreds of thousands of women have undergone the knife to improve their own physiognomy and frame, most remarkably their breasts.

Be warned, as they say on the television news channels: some of what follows may be offensive, shocking, or just downright crazy, and make you close your eyes and legs. Parental guidance is definitely advised.

Let's start with three prescription medicines that pre-date Viagra and were in use in the West and other parts of the world, including Asia: Caverject, Edex, and Muse, all used to treat male impotence. The first two were administered by hypodermic injection, a system described in excruciating detail by David Friedman in *Esquire* magazine in September 1997 in an article titled "Are You Man Enough to Handle a Four-Hour Erection?" Friedman called impotence a "growth industry"—it's difficult not to pun recklessly when talking about this—pointing out (see what I mean?) that "injection therapy, as I now know from experience, works whether you're aroused or not. Assuming the dosage is adequate and the shot has been properly administered, the penis must follow orders. The ultimate male fantasy has come true: a penis that's hard on demand, hard after orgasm, hard for hours, hard enough to satisfy the most demanding woman. Even a bunch of them."

The way such pharmaceutical wonders were administered was by direct hypodermic injection, not into an arm or buttock, something most men found acceptable if not especially welcome, but right into the flaccid penis. This was done just before sex was anticipated and because response was almost immediate, a syringe came with the prescription and patients were shown how to inject themselves. No need, after all, to waste a perfectly good hard-on while stuck in traffic on the way home from the doctor's office.

The third of these drugs, Muse, was taken as a small suppository inserted into the *urethra* by a plastic plunger that Friedman said resembled a Pez candy dispenser. As Dave Barry says about so many things, I'm not making this up.

Believe it or not, as many as a million men, most of them in the U.S., along with an unknown number in Asia, were treated with these drugs in 1996 and 1997. More than 350,000 men took the Pez cure alone during the first six months it was publicly available. Then came Viagra and after that, no one heard much about prescription injections and urethral suppositories again. Which couldn't have been much of a surprise.

Injections of another type, aimed at more permanent change, have found a larger audience in Asia, as, for example, when fat cells from elsewhere in the body were harvested by a procedure called liposuction and injected below the skin surface of the penis to increase girth. (But not length; nor can the head, or glans, be enlarged.) Silicone and collagen were used for the same purpose—and inserted into the ball sac as well—but none of these substances has been all that popular, especially since silicone was banned in the West from use in breast implants. Side effects can be horrendous, the result a sight to applaud, but elasticity like ferro cement.

Non-prescription injections are another thing. Consider this story from *The Nation*, one of Bangkok's English language dailies, dated May 16, 2005, when it was reported that young men in Ayutthaya, better known for its ancient, conical religious monuments, were injecting their penises with extra virgin olive oil and beta "agonist," a chemical used to redden meat.

This practice may have been "Doctor Tested & Approved" (quoting a dubious website advertisement), but Dr. Chatri Banchuin, director-general of Thailand's Department of Medical Services, said that instead of making what is sometimes called a King Naga (so called for the snake god) merely bigger, the oil could build up in the penis, causing swelling, inflammation and abscesses.

Many other substances have been injected directly into the Asian penis or scrotum, including silicone, collagen, mineral oil, KY Jelly, and Vaseline. This can cause enormous increases in girth of the penis and capacity of the scrotal sack—as much as several hundred percent—but it is effectively irreversible and may have side effects including loss of sensation, inability to perform penetrative intercourse, scarring, and deformation.

Another practice found mainly in Indonesia and South Asia—and more popular here than anywhere else in the world, apparently—is called genital beading, a body modification that calls for the implantation of foreign objects beneath the surface of the penile skin. Usually, stainless steel, titanium, or Teflon beads are used but even small pebbles will do. Sometimes this is called pearling, after the Yakuza practice of implanting pearls, usually while in prison, one pearl for each year of incarceration. Imagine it. Some of those guys get life sentences.

A story in the *Malay Mail* in August 1994 quoted an unidentified urologist in Kuala Lumpur as saying he'd treated patients with nodules who wanted them removed when the penis became infected and inflamed. The afternoon tabloid said it was following up on a case involving a prostitute who had been fined $40 for hitting her client with a broom after refusing to accept his ball-bearing-laden penis. She told the court that it wasn't an uncommon practice and that she had encountered clients with up to eight objects buried beneath the skin.

Not so long ago, virtually all such body modifications were self-administered. (Accompanied by or following, perhaps, a large quantity of self-administered alcohol.) Nowadays, with the popularity of body piercing—usually on the face, but increasingly involving the nipples and genitals—the service is offered by numerous Asian tattoo parlors.

More common today is what is called penile enhancement surgery, a catch-all phrase that includes a simple severing of the suspensory ligaments at the top and base of the penile shaft, allowing that part of the cock normally "inside" the body to "fall" away, shifting part of the "root" outside. This can result in significantly greater length, up to five centimeters (two inches) in rare cases. What this means, though, is that while the cock still further elongates and stiffens as blow flow occurs, it no longer becomes truly erect, but angles downward.

One physician I talked to compared the difference to a Concorde taking off and a Concorde landing. Another said, "Before the operation, you could hang a heavy jacket on your hard-on, after it maybe your shirt."

Still another surgical procedure, suggested for men suffering from complete impotency, replaced the two *corpora cavernosa* with inflatable implants. This also required an implanted pump in the groin that could be manipulated by hand, sort of like inflating a beach toy with a bellows.

This surgery is extremely fashionable in the West, becoming what journalists inevitably called a "growth industry" in the early 1990s, when most Asian men went to Australia for the big cut. What is interesting is that most of the innovators in the U.S. studied with a penis-lengthening innovator by the name of—I kid you not—Dr. Long Daochou of Wuhan, in central China.

It was the plight of a young accountant whose cock was bitten off by a dog that first drew Dr. Long to the field. An only son, the twenty-two year old patient was under pressure to marry and produce an heir. Dr. Long operated and the unlucky accountant fathered a daughter. That was in 1984. Thousands of operations followed, with acclaim by the Chinese news agency Xinhua. But now he is largely unknown.

So, too, the countless cosmetic surgeons in Asia who now regard breast enhancement surgery, or augmentation mammoplasty, their bread and butter.

When I moved to Thailand in 1993, virtually all Asian women had small breasts. That is to say, "natural" breasts, unaltered by silicone and saline, as was so pervasive in parts of the West. Today, as cosmetic surgery drives much of what is called "medical tourism" in Asia, not only are foreign women flying to Bangkok, Singapore, Hong Kong, Taipei, and Tokyo for a "boob job," but so, too, are their Asian sisters queuing to have small (or large), round and contoured medical-grade sacs containing saline surgically implanted in their chests.

As was the case with penis enlargement, the story of breast implants is believed to have begun in Asia, when Japanese prostitutes in the 1940s injected substances like paraffin or surgically implanted sponge, believing this made them more attractive to American GIs serving in the occupation forces following World War Two.

In the time since, procedures have changed radically. Where once, surgical entry was made beneath the breast or on the perimeter of the areola, usually leaving a visible scar, now the incisions are small and placed so that scarring is minimal, perhaps through the woman's armpit. The surgeon then cuts a path through the tissue and a pocket is created for the implant. In more extreme augmentation, the nipple may be repositioned, adjusting for cleavage and creating a new crease under the breast, accompanied by a "breast lift" so that everything ends up in the right place. Pre-filled implants may be used or, increasingly now, the doc will use a syringe to fill an empty one to the predetermined size with saline through a valve.

It should be mentioned that there may be, proportionately, fewer crackpots and fraudsters out there performing surgery than there are selling so-called "aphrodisiacs." But they are there, and in number. The field of cosmetic surgery is, in many Asian countries, unregulated and where there are laws, they often go unenforced. Street clinics sometimes deliver disaster; one poor woman in Thailand not long ago had to have condoms filled with who knows what removed from her chest when infection occurred.

My advice is to skip surgery when all that's desired is more. If you really do have ill-formed or damaged breasts or genitals, by all means see a certified expert in the field of reconstructive surgery. Otherwise, try to find happiness with what you've got.

Which reminds me of the man who answered an advertisement for a penis enlarger and received in the mail a cheap magnifying glass.

It worked, didn't it?

Afterword
Things That Work

Constantly I encountered two things in my search for aphrodisiacs that worked yet inevitably got in the way.

One was that so little clinical examination had been carried out under "acceptable" laboratory conditions. By the time researchers finally were finding that some foods, herbs, and other supplements did stimulate production of hormones or other chemicals that affected the libido, they still didn't know if those chemicals were produced in sufficient quantity for anyone to really know the difference. To be fair to those scientific explorers, one of the reasons there isn't much hard research in the area is that libido is a difficult thing to study.

So the "facts" are hard to pin down. Still, it does appear that some of what's been praised for centuries does offer more than mere promise. As so many of my teachers long ago said at the end of a semester: let's review.

Even the most casual reader will have noticed that most of the stuff claimed to have aphrodisiacal qualities wouldn't even make a good cup of tea. This has been true through the ages, and not just in Asia, but everywhere.

It should also have been clear that many of the substances, both animal and vegetable, were often consumed for reasons other than increased sexual prowess. Many of these also promised overall good health and long life, or a way to fight off cancer or flatulence, so those individuals who paid good money for the potions or pills or expensive bowls of soup could tell themselves that even if it didn't make them Asia's answer to Warren Beatty, it served them in other ways.

Okay, let's get down to the nitty-gritty. Putting aside the placebo effect, which apparently has real if mysterious effect but obviously is not anything you can count on, let's first look back at some of the herbs and plants touted in the millennia-old medical systems found in China, India, and elsewhere. One of the most important things to note is that no quick fixes were promised: if you want results, you have to consume the stuff for an extended period of time...and it wouldn't hurt any if you stopped drinking and smoking, started exercising, reduced stress, and improved your diet. The guy who gulped a *jamu* tonic in Jakarta on his way into a brothel may think it did some good—and therefore maybe it did, through the placebo effect—but that isn't the way *jamu* works. Whether you're trying to maintain or restore balance between *yin* and *yang* or your *doshas* or whatever, balance and commitment are as important as the ingredients consumed.

Bottom line: those who adhere to the shock tactics of Western medicine may remain skeptical. The developed world is embracing the holistic approach to health rapidly, but as even Carroll Dunham, the "Dr. Ruth of the Himalayas" and a true believer, admits, there is an alarming absence of clinical testing that is acceptable in the West. She and others like her, including a majority of the people in some of the most populous countries on earth, will continue to credit the thousands of years of medical history in Asia as something too good to be ignored, as something that for them really works.

All that said, there are several substances that time seems to favor, even amongst non-believers. Opium and marijuana are two, especially the latter. And any botanical ingredient that stimulates blood flow, any product that contains zinc or amino acids, and anything that produces an itchiness in the genital area probably contributes to the pleasure of sex if taken in reasonable quantities.

The same thing can be said about alcohol and many of the chemicals, especially the modern ED drugs, along with the counterfeit copies, but also the illegal ones such as Ecstasy, amphetamines, and poppers.

There's more. Most lubricants do precisely what they're supposed to, with or without camphor and other stimulants added. Massage is nearly always effective, as it arouses the natural endomorphins or feels good because its been a long time since you've felt a friendly touch on what is, after all, the largest organ in the body with the most nerve endings, the skin.

Many of the mechanical devices do the job, as well, although much of the workmanship is shoddy and they're usually overpriced. For instance, dildos and vibrators perform admirably, often better than most men. Cock rings usually deliver a longer, harder erection for men and anal beads may offer him or his partner an added kick.

Pornography can be a turn-on, for those who enjoy it, for women as well as men. And in Asia, unlike in the West, when it's bootlegged it's affordable.

Music can provide a nice prelude and an exciting accompaniment.

And surgery can make you bigger where you want to be bigger. Or turn you into the opposite sex.

A little caring, loving attention doesn't hurt, either. And usually it will go a lot further than all the stuff we'd done to ourselves in its absence and consumed along the way.

This book is different from most books about aphrodisiacs in that most usually praise or damn—and rarely both—and the vast majority are so flattering or, hidden in what the authors think is "objectivity," they are no more helpful than the so-called aphrodisiacs themselves.

And they're all so damned serious. I've tried to have fun with the "remedies" because, after all, that's a large part of what sex is all about: having fun. So my best advice is to have fun, try not to spend too much money, and don't get your hopes up, because that's all that may come up in the end.